STUBBORN BELLY FAT REMOVER

The Ultimate Abdominal Architect for a Balanced Body

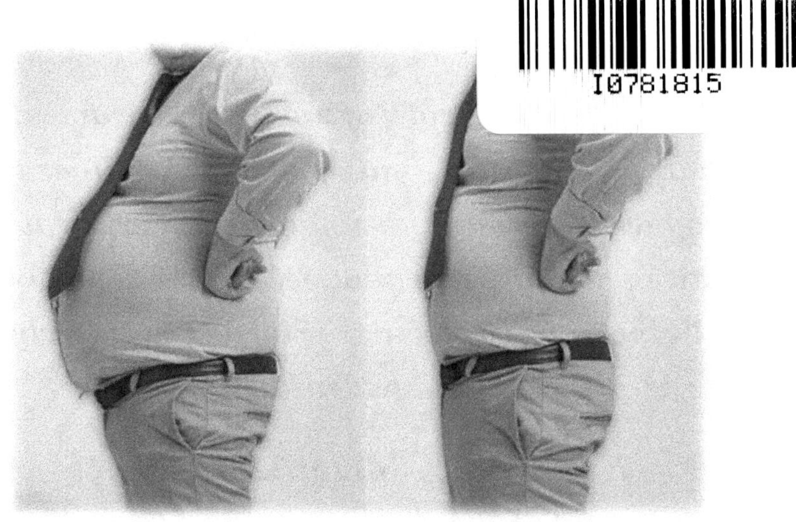

MELISSA J. LEVEY

Copyright Page

© 2024 [**MELISSA J. LEVEY**]

Cover design by [**MELISSA J. LEVEY**]

Published by [**MELISSA J. LEVEY**]

PREFACE

Imagine having to deal with the weight of frustration every morning when you glance in the mirror and see that obstinate tummy fat that never seems to go away. For 38-year-old Seattle software developer Mark Thompson, this was life. Mark had tried everything from bogus detoxes to exercise regimens to diets. Nothing seemed to work. The abdominal fat affected his confidence, health, and general happiness like an unwanted visitor.

It's not just Mark who struggles. Among the hardest and most prevalent problems millions of people worldwide deal with is belly obesity. Excess belly fat has significant health risks like heart disease, diabetes, and metabolic problems; it's not just about looks. Gaining knowledge about and conquering this problem calls for a thorough and long-term strategy rather than only a band-aid solution.

Mark's path started off frustrating but ended triumphant. One day he happened into a book called "Stubborn Belly Fat Remover" while perusing a neighborhood bookshop. Distressed for a solution and intrigued by its claims, he chose to give it a shot. Nothing he had attempted previously compared to the book. It gave more than simply short cuts; it gave a comprehensive explanation of the reasons belly fat is so tenacious and how to deal with it.

For the following several months, Mark assiduously adhered to the tactics outlined in the book. He studied about the biology of belly fat, the value of a well-balanced diet, and the kinds of activities that are especially designed to reduce belly fat. Having learned how stress and sleep affected his weight, he included doable advice to control these variables. His exploration of the psychological components of weight loss also served to keep him focused and motivated.

Incredible were the outcomes. Mark not only shed the years-long belly fat, but he also acquired renewed confidence and vigor. Though it took dedication, tolerance, and a readiness to adapt, his path was not without its rewards. Mark showed his friends and family that anyone can reach their health objectives with the correct information and attitude by transforming himself.

This book is your road map to success if you've been fighting resistant belly fat and feel like nothing is working. More than simply a book, "Stubborn Belly Fat Remover" is an all-inclusive manual meant to help you recognize and overcome the challenges in your way. Following the methods and doable suggestions in these pages, you may change your body and take back your health.

Give up letting irritation stop you. Take the first step towards a healthier, happier you. Explore "Stubborn Belly Fat Remover" to learn the strategies you need to at last get the outcomes you've been hoping for. Your path to a more confident, fitter you begin right now. Ready to make a change, Start now.

Comprehending Stubborn Belly Fat

The Science

Sometimes the most annoying and obstinate kind of fat, belly fat is more than just a surface-level problem. It stands for a major risk factor for a number of medical disorders. Knowing the basic science of belly fat is essential to addressing this problem successfully.

Belly Fat Types

Subcutaneous fat and visceral fat are the two primary categories into which belly fat falls.

- ***Subcutaneous Fat***: Just under the skin is this fat. It's the sort you can pinch with your fingertips and, in general, is less bad for you than visceral fat. Although it could not be very attractive visually, it is not very harmful to health.

- ***Fat Visceral***: Deep within the abdominal cavity, around internal organs like the pancreas, intestines, and liver, is where this kind of fat stores. Because visceral fat is metabolically active, it releases a variety of chemicals that can aggravate inflammation and tamper with hormone levels. It is intimately related to medical conditions including metabolic syndrome, type 2 diabetes, and cardiovascular disease.

The Part Hormones Play

Abdominal fat builds up and is distributed mostly in response to hormones. Important hormones consist on

Insulin: Blood sugar levels are helped to be regulated by this hormone. Insulin spikes from a diet heavy in refined sugars and carbohydrates, which encourages fat storage, especially around the abdomen.

- ***Cortisol***: Often referred to as the stress hormone, cortisol is produced in reaction to tension. Prolonged high levels of cortisol brought on by chronic stress might heighten hunger and promote the storage of belly fat.
- ***Ghrelin and Leptin***: These hormones control when you're hungry and full. Production of leptin by fat cells alerts the brain to fullness. Ghrelin, however, increases appetite. Overeating and weight gain may result from imbalances in these hormones.

Genetic Contributor

Where your body accumulates fat is also mostly determined by heredity. Some individuals are genetically prone to store fat in their abdomens. Although your genes cannot be changed, knowing this aspect can enable you to use more focused methods to fight belly obesity.

Belly fat and metabolism

Our metabolism naturally slows with age, which makes weight gain simpler and weight loss more difficult, particularly around the abdomen. Among the elements affecting metabolic rate are

- **Mass of Muscles**: Even while asleep, muscle tissue consumes more calories than fat tissue. The tendency of muscular mass to decline with age can slow down metabolism.
- **Regular exercise**: Increases muscle mass and encourages effective energy usage, which increases metabolism.
- **The diet**: You metabolic rate is influenced by the kinds and amounts of food you eat. More so than diets heavy in fats or carbs, diets strong in protein can boost metabolism.

Knowing how these elements interact intricately is essential to creating workable plans to fight obstinate abdominal fat.

Belly fat loss is infamously hard, and a number of things go into it.

Fat Cell Behavior

Diverse regions of the body have diverse behaviors from their fat cells. Because the abdominal fat cells are more metabolically active and have a larger density of cortisol receptors, they are more prone to accumulate fat when cortisol levels are high. Furthermore, compared to beta-2 adrenergic receptors, alpha-2 adrenergic receptors are more abundant in cells of the belly fat. The inability to break down fat in these locations is exacerbated by alpha-2 receptors.

Insulin Resistance

An often occurring problem linked to belly obesity is insulin resistance. The pancreas increases insulin production to make up for cells in the body becoming less sensitive to it. Particularly in the abdomen, high insulin levels encourage fat storage. This starts a vicious circle in which more belly fat causes more insulin resistance, which raises insulin resistance and so causes more belly fat.

Critical

Known to be inflammatory agents, visceral fat produces cytokines. Further complicating attempts at weight loss, these cytokines can impede the body's capacity to control insulin and may even lead to chronic inflammation. Furthermore complicating weight loss is inflammation's promotion of a state of ongoing stress in the body, which raises cortisol levels.

Nutritional Considerations

Many people use diet to unintentionally undermine their attempts to lose weight. Refined sugar and carbohydrate intakes can cause insulin and blood sugar increases that encourage fat storage. It can also be more difficult to sustain a calorie deficit needed for weight loss when one consumes more calories and feels less satisfied on diets heavy in processed foods, bad fats, and sugary drinks.

Physical Inactivity

Sitting a lot of the time adds a lot to abdominal fat buildup. Little exercise lowers muscle mass, slows metabolism, and burns fewer calories. Building muscle, which can increase metabolism and encourage more efficient fat reduction, is just as important as burning calories during regular exercise.

Sleep and Stress

Unbelievably important but sometimes disregarded causes of abdominal fat buildup include chronic stress and sleep deprivation. Cortisol, a hormone raised by stress, can make one hungrier and more likely to crave high-calorie foods. Unhealthy sleep throws off the chemicals that control hunger, raising ghrelin (which increases appetite) and lowering leptin (which indicates fullness). Especially in the waist, this hormonal imbalance can cause overeating and weight gain.

AGE

Ageing is linked, as was already indicated, to a normal loss in metabolic rate and muscular mass. As we age, hormonal changes like lower levels of sex hormones and growth hormone can lead to more fat accumulation and trouble shedding abdominal fat.

Agenda

Approaching this prevalent issue requires first understanding the science underlying abdominal fat and the reasons why it is difficult to reduce. One way to create a healthier body is to address the biochemical, hormonal, genetic, and behavioral elements that lead to belly obesity. We'll go over thorough plans in the upcoming chapters that include exercise, food, lifestyle modifications, and psychological elements to help you permanently lose stubborn belly fat.

Benefits of Stubborn Belly Fat Remover

> ### *Comprehensive coverage of all aspects of belly fat removal*
> Stubborn Belly Fat Remover delves deeply into all aspects of belly fat reduction, leaving no stone untouched. From the fundamental biology of belly fat to the most recent medicinal and surgical procedures, every detail is thoroughly explored to provide readers a thorough understanding of the subject.

> ### *Scientific Approach Using Evidence-Based Information*
> Stubborn Belly Fat Remover is based on scientific research and evidence-based techniques, providing readers with credible and trustworthy information that is supported by scientific rigor. By synthesizing findings from peer-reviewed studies, clinical trials, and expert consensus, the book ensures that readers

get accurate and up-to-date information on effective fat loss procedures.

➢ ***Useful Tips on Nutrition, Exercise, and Lifestyle Changes***
Beyond theoretical information, "Stubborn Belly Fat Remover" provides readers with real guidance and solutions to apply in their daily lives. Whether it's advice on improving food habits, creating efficient training routines, or implementing stress management techniques, the book enables readers to make practical changes that support their fat loss goals.

➢ ***Including Psychological Factors and Motivational Strategies***
Recognizing the critical role of psychological elements in successful fat loss, the book discusses the significance of mindset, motivation, and behavior change. By digging into topics such as emotional eating, body image concerns, and goal planning, Stubborn Belly Fat Remover offers a reader essential insights and tactics for overcoming mental hurdles and cultivating a positive attitude.

➢ ***Real-life Success Stories to Motivate Readers***
Drawing inspiration from real-life success stories, "Stubborn Belly Fat Remover" gives readers hope and encouragement by highlighting people who have undergone incredible transformations. These inspiring stories serve as powerful examples of what is possible with dedication, determination, and the correct tools, encouraging readers to embark on their own fat reduction path with confidence.

> ### *A Step-by-Step Guide for Creating a Personalized Plan*
>
> The book takes readers step by step through the process of establishing a personalized fat reduction strategy, ensuring that individual needs, preferences, and goals are considered. From examining beginning points to setting realistic objectives and tracking progress, each aspect of the trip is meticulously planned, empowering readers to take control of their health and well-being.

> ### *Comprehensive Resources for Additional Support and Learning*
>
> Stubborn Belly Fat Remover extends beyond the book's pages, offering readers a wealth of additional assistance and information. Readers get access to a plethora of resources to support their fat reduction journey and improve their knowledge and skills, including online groups and recommended reading as well as expert coaching from nutritionists and personal trainers.

Conclusion

In "Stubborn Belly Fat Remover," readers are given a comprehensive, scientifically grounded, and practical guide to achieving long-term fat removal and restoring their health and vigor. By addressing all areas of belly fat removal, presenting evidence-based information and practical advice, and providing resources for additional support and study, the book enables readers to embark on a transforming journey towards a healthier, happier living.

Stubborn Belly Fat Remover is an invaluable resource for anyone looking to conquer stubborn belly fat and achieve their fat loss goals.

Cons of Stubborn Belly Fat Remover

1. *May be overwhelming due to the amount of information*

While "Stubborn Belly Fat Remover" aims to give complete coverage of fat loss strategies, the sheer number of material presented in its pages may be overwhelming for some readers. The amount of scientific research, practical guidance, and case studies may cause information overload, making it difficult for readers to understand and implement all of the knowledge efficiently.

2. *Requires commitment and time to read through and implement strategies.*

To achieve fat loss, you must be committed, dedicated, and consistent in executing the tactics given in the book. However, some readers may struggle to devote the necessary time and effort to thoroughly reading the book and actively implementing the recommended tactics in their daily life. As a result, adherence to the program may be jeopardized, impeding the achievement of desired fat reduction results.

3. *Some chapters may not be relevant to everyone (e.g. medical interventions).*

While Stubborn Belly Fat Remover strives to provide a wide range of fat loss methods, not all chapters may be relevant to each reader. For example, people who are primarily concerned with lifestyle changes may find chapters on medical procedures less relevant to their requirements. This lack of relevance may reduce the total value of the work for certain readers, leading to disengagement or irritation.

4. *The scientific content may be complex for those without a background in health or science.*

Despite efforts to convey scientific material in an understandable manner, some readers with no background in health or science may struggle to comprehend the complexity of the scientific content presented in "Stubborn Belly Fat Remover." Individuals who are unfamiliar with analyzing scientific literature may find technical words, study findings, and physiological explanations difficult to understand, potentially leading to confusion or disinterest.

Mitigation Strategies

To remedy these shortcomings and improve the overall reader experience, Stubborn Belly Fat Remover might consider using the following mitigating strategies:

1. *Streamlining Information*: Simplify and compress difficult topics to avoid overwhelming readers with too much information. Focus on delivering essential lessons and actionable strategies in a clear and simple manner.

2. ***Provide Summaries and Action Plans***: give summaries at the end of each chapter to highlight key ideas and give readers with specific steps for implementing the strategies covered. These summaries can be used as short reference guides for readers who want to review important material without having to read complete chapters.

3. ***Customizing information***: Tailor the information to meet readers' different requirements and preferences by providing customizable pathways or recommendations based on personal goals, interests, and backgrounds. This method allows readers to focus on the chapters and strategies that are most relevant to their specific situations.

4. ***Enhancing Accessibility***: Use visual aids, illustrations, and practical examples to supplement written content and improve comprehension for readers from various backgrounds. Additionally, provide glossaries, footnotes, or online resources to help readers understand technical vocabulary and navigate scientific concepts.

By using these mitigation measures, "*Stubborn Belly Fat Remover*" can address potential flaws and improve the reader experience, ensuring that the book stays accessible, interesting, and beneficial for anyone looking to achieve long-term fat removal and increased health and well-being.

Belly Fat Biology

Belly Fat Types: [Visceral vs. Subcutaneous]

Though many individuals worry about belly fat, not all belly fat is made equal. Creating successful tactics to fight belly fat requires an understanding of the several kinds and their unique traits. Explored in this chapter are the functions, hazards, and responses to food and exercise of the two main forms of belly fat: visceral and subcutaneous fat.

Fat under the Skin

Fat that is just under the skin is called subcutaneous fat. Most usually seen in the abdomen, thighs, and buttocks, it is the fat you can pinch between your fingers.

- **Functionality**: It serves as an energy reserve, giving the body fuel when it is short on calories.

- **Insulation**: It lowers heat loss, which helps to insulate the body and regulate body temperature.

- **Protective measures**: It shields and cushions underlying muscles and organs from injury.

Consequences for Health

Though less dangerous than visceral fat, subcutaneous fat can nonetheless cause health issues in excess:

- ***Metabolic Health***: Insulin resistance diabetes are among the metabolic problems linked to high amounts of subcutaneous fat.
- ***Inflammation***: It can generate inflammatory markers, which feeds the body's chronic inflammation.
- ***Aesthetics***: Overabundance of subcutaneous fat can have an impact on self-esteem and attractiveness.

The Diet and Exercise Response

Conventional weight-loss methods work effectively on subcutaneous fat:

- ***Diet***: Lowering total calorie intake and following a balanced diet high in complex carbs, lean proteins, healthy fats, and whole foods can help lower subcutaneous fat.
- ***Exercise***: Strength training along with aerobic exercise like swimming, cycling, and jogging can successfully reduce subcutaneous fat levels.

Fat Visceral

Term and Place

Storing itself far within the abdominal cavity, visceral fat envelops important organs like the pancreas, liver, and intestines. It cannot be pinched and is not visible like subcutaneous fat.

- ***Function***: More directly linked to negative health impacts, visceral fat has fewer advantages
- ***Hormonal Activity***: Metabolically active, it releases a range of hormones and inflammatory chemicals that might interfere with regular body processes.
- ***The Risk Factor***: Many major medical disorders, such as type 2 diabetes, cardiovascular disease, and some malignancies, are significantly increased by it.

Consequences for Health

Health hazards from visceral fat are higher than those from subcutaneous fat:

Its impact on blood pressure and cholesterol levels as well as its close proximity to important organs raises the risk of heart disease and stroke.

The precursor to type 2 diabetes, insulin resistance, is closely associated with visceral fat.

- ***Inflammation***: Cytokines it produces can lead to chronic inflammation and aggravate metabolic problems even further.
- ***Fatty Liver Disease***: Non-alcoholic fatty liver disease, which can lead to liver cirrhosis and failure, is linked with excess visceral fat.

The Diet and Exercise Response

Although it can be harder to remove visceral fat, it is quite sensitive to some lifestyle modifications:

- ***Diet***: Visceral fat can be greatly decreased by a diet strong in fiber, lean proteins, and healthy fats and low in processed sweets. Especially beneficial is a Mediterranean diet high in fruits, vegetables, whole grains, and good fats.
- ***Exercise***: Regular cardiovascular exercise and High-Intensity Interval Training (HIIT) work especially well to lower visceral fat. Muscle mass increases from strength training also promote metabolism and help with fat loss.
- ***Reduction of Stress***: Stress reduction strategies include yoga, meditation, and enough sleep are essential since stress raises cortisol levels, which encourage the development of visceral fat.

The Interplay of Visceral and Subcutaneous Fat

Deviations in Metabolism

Though both kinds of fat are related to metabolic health, because of its location and hormonal activity, visceral fat is more strongly associated with metabolic diseases. More serious health effects than with subcutaneous fat can result from the chemicals generated by visceral fat interfering with insulin signaling and lipid metabolism.

- ***Assessment and Measuring***: BMI (body mass index) Though it cannot differentiate between visceral and subcutaneous fat, BMI can give a broad estimate of body fat.
- ***Circumference of the Waist***: Assessing visceral fat is made easier with this test. More than 40 inches for males and 35 inches for women is a waist circumference that indicates extra visceral fat and higher health risks.
- ***Imaging Methodologies***: Though they are expensive and not widely available outside of clinical settings, advanced techniques like MRI and CT scans can assess visceral fat with great accuracy.

Gender Variations

Owing to hormonal differences, men and women often store fat differently:

- ***Men***: Those with an "apple-shaped" body are more prone to gain visceral fat.
- ***Women***: Often have a "pear-shaped" figure because they retain more subcutaneous fat, especially around the hips and thighs. Because to hormonal changes, postmenopausal women may, nevertheless, accumulate more visceral fat.

Biological

Furthermore influencing fat distribution are genetic elements. Adopting customized fat reduction plans depending on individual risk factors and body composition is essential because some people are genetically predisposed to retain more visceral fat.

Synopsis

For efficient weight control and health enhancement, one must know the distinctions between visceral and subcutaneous fat. Even if subcutaneous fat has several energy-storage and defensive purposes, too much of it might cause health problems. But because it's so close to important organs and helps to cause metabolic problems, visceral fat is more dangerous to health.

Knowing the different qualities and effects on health of these two fat kinds will help you customize your lifestyle, diet, and exercise regimen to more successfully target and decrease belly fat. This book's later chapters will offer thorough instructions on how to put these tactics into practice, enabling you to build a stronger, leaner, and more vibrant body.

Belly Fat Hormonal Factors

In controlling the distribution of body fat, especially the buildup of belly fat, hormones are essential. Knowledge of the hormonal variables affecting belly fat might help one better control and minimize it. The major hormones involved in fat metabolism and storage are discussed in this chapter along with how they particularly impact abdominal fat.

Insulin and Function within the Body

The pancreatic hormone insulin controls blood sugar levels. It enables circulatory glucose absorption by cells for storage as fat or usage as energy.

- **Insulin Resistance**: The body makes extra insulin to make up for cells that lose their sensitivity to it. Especially in the abdomen, high insulin levels encourage fat storage. Insulin resistance, a prelude to type 2 diabetes, is intimately related to the buildup of visceral fat.
- **Affect of Diet**: Insulin resistance and the development of belly fat can be exacerbated by regular insulin spikes brought on by diets heavy in refined

sugars and carbs. Low-glycemic meals and carbohydrate intake management can help lessen these effects.

Nor epinephrine and Function within the Body

One hormone the adrenal glands release in reaction to stress is cortisol. Among the many body processes it is essential to include metabolism, the immune system, and stress control.

The effect on belly fat with Stress and fat storage

Long-term high cortisol levels brought on by chronic stress might heighten hunger and sugar- and calorie-hungry cravings. Especially around the abdomen, this behavior encourages fat storage.

Metabolic Impact: Inhibiting insulin action, high cortisol levels can also exacerbate insulin resistance and the buildup of belly fat.

Lifestyle Techniques: Reduced cortisol levels and a decreased propensity to accumulate fat in the abdomen can be achieved with stress management strategies including mindfulness, meditation, and regular exercise.

Ghrelin and Leptin

Leptin

Function within the Body

Prod by fat cells, leptin alerts the brain to control energy balance and hunger. It basically alerts your brain to the point at which you should stop eating.

- **Impact on Belly Fat**: Leptin Resistance Low body fat people may develop leptin resistance, a disorder in which the brain becomes less responsive to the hormone. Overeating and ongoing hunger follow from this, which adds to the accumulation of fat—including belly fat.
- **Controlling Weigh**: Lowering weight can raise leptin sensitivity. Mainstays of leptin homeostasis and prevention of belly fat buildup are a balanced diet high in healthy foods and regular exercise.

Ghrelin

Function within the Body

Appetite-stimulating hormone ghrelin is made in the stomach. It is essential to starting meals since it tells the brain to feel hungry.

Impact on Belly Fat Increased Appetite: Ghrelin levels above normal might cause overeating and increased hunger, which can increase weight growth and belly fat.

The Sleep Connection: Decreased leptin and higher ghrelin levels linked to poor sleep create a hormonal milieu that encourages fat storage and increased appetite. Sustaining normal ghrelin levels requires getting enough good sleep.

Estrogen

Function within the Body

Primary female sex hormone estrogen controls a number of processes, such as fat distribution, bone density, and reproductive health.

- ***The Affect on Belly Fat***: Because estrogen levels drop after menopause, fat might move from the hips and thighs to the abdomen. This change is one factor in postmenopausal women's higher visceral fat levels.
- ***HRT or hormone replacement treatment***: Though there are possible hazards, HRT should be used carefully and under medical supervision to help lessen some of the symptoms of lowering estrogen levels.

Testosterone

Function within the Body

A key hormone of male sex, testosterone affects metabolism generally, distribution of fat, and muscle mass.

- ***Age-Related Decline***: Effect on Belly Fat When testosterone levels naturally drop as men age, body fat—especially visceral fat—increases and muscle mass falls.
- ***Increasing Testosterone Levels***: Belly fat can be reduced and testosterone levels increased with resistance training, a sufficient protein diet, and good weight maintenance.

Belly fat distribution and genetics

Genetics also significantly affects where and how your body stores fat, even if hormones play a major influence in fat distribution. You can more successfully customize your weight control techniques if you are aware of the hereditary variables affecting belly fat.

The Genetic Predisposition

- ***Genetic Influence***: Certain individuals are more prone to store fat in their abdomens, while others may store it in their hips, thighs, or other places.
- ***History of the Family***: You might be destined to accumulate fat in your abdomen if obesity or central obesity—fat buildup in the belly—runs in your family.

- ***Key Genes Involved***: Higher body fat and an increased risk of obesity are linked with variations in the FTO gene. People with particular FTO gene variations typically have more appetites and less satiety, which increases calorie intake and fat storage.
- ***Gene MC4R***: Energy balance and appetite regulation are functions of the MC4R gene. Increased appetite , a propensity to weight gain and the buildup of abdominal fat can result from mutations in this gene.

Inheritance

Environmental Interactions

Changes in gene expression brought on by environmental influences are referred to as epigenetic, not modifications in the genetic code per such. How your genes are expressed can be influenced by lifestyle choices including nutrition, exercise, and stress.

- ***Nutritional Epigenetic:*** Changes in gene expression brought on by poor diet can encourage obesity and fat storage. On the other hand, a good diet lowers the chance of abdominal fat buildup by favorably affecting gene expression.
- ***Physical Activity and Genetics***: Frequent physical activity can help lower abdominal fat and enhance metabolic health generally by changing the expression of genes associated to fat metabolism and storage.

Gender Disparities

- ***Patterns of Fat Distribution***: Men the "apple-shaped" physique that results from men's propensity to retain fat in the abdomen region. Greater levels of visceral fat, which is more dangerous for health, affect this pattern.
- ***Femmes***: Usually storing fat in the hips, thighs, and buttocks, women have a "pear-shaped" physique. But hormonal changes brought on by menopause can cause fat storage to go to the abdomen.
- ***Genetic Variability***: Men and women express some fat-distributing genes differently. Where fat is kept in the body is determined, for instance, in part by genes linked to androgen receptors and estrogen.

Ethnic and Racial Disparities

Diverse Genetics

Genetic variances across races and ethnicities can also affect the distribution of fat

- ***African origin***: The tendency of people of African origin to accumulate subcutaneous fat instead of visceral fat may affect the hazards to general health.
- ***Asian Descent***: Those of Asian heritage are more likely to accumulate visceral fat, even at lower body weights, which raises their risk of metabolic disorders.

- ***Caucasian Descent***: Although their patterns of fat storage can be greatly impacted by lifestyle choices, people of Caucasian descent may have a more evenly distributed subcutaneous and visceral fat.

Synopsis

Particularly in the abdominal region, the interaction between hormones and heredity is quite important in shaping the fat distribution. Knowing these things will help you to develop more individualized and successful belly fat-fighting tactics. Hormonal balance can be attained via nutrition, exercise, stress reduction, and enough sleep; understanding hereditary predispositions can also assist establish reasonable expectations and goals.

The chapters that follow will look at doable methods for reducing belly fat, including diet, exercise, lifestyle modifications, and psychological techniques to help you get and stay in better physical shape. With the integration of this information, you may create a thorough plan catered to your particular hormonal and genetic profile, therefore maximizing your efforts to lose belly fat and enhance general health.

Diet and Insulin Resistance

The distribution of body fat—including the buildup of belly fat—is mostly determined by nutrition. Your body retains fat in part because of the kinds of foods you eat, when you eat, and how many calories you consume overall. Making wise decisions to control and effectively reduce belly fat can be facilitated by knowing how various food elements contribute to it.

The Part Diet Plays in Fat Buildup

- ***Caloric Balance -Excess Energy***: The extra calories your body stores as fat are those you consume more of what it requires. Increases in visceral and subcutaneous fat may result from this excess.
- ***Inadequate Energy Supply***: Less calories than your body needs, on the other hand, result in fat reduction. Reducing abdominal fat requires food and exercise to provide a modest calorie deficit.
- ***Nutrient Content***: Diets heavy in whole foods like vegetables, fruits, lean meats, and whole grains—offer vital nutrients and fiber that help regulate metabolism and lower abdominal fat. By contrast, processed diets heavy in refined grains, bad fats, and added sugars might encourage the buildup of fat, especially in the abdomen.

- ***TIME of Meal***: Blood sugar levels can be controlled and overeating can be avoided by eating smaller, more frequent meals. Additionally, eating lighter meals in the evening and bigger meals earlier in the day supports more efficient fat metabolism by lining up with the body's natural metabolic rhythms.
- ***Short Term Fasting***: With this dietary plan, eating and fasting times are interchanged. Intermittent fasting has been linked in some research to increased insulin sensitivity, decreased visceral fat, and general fat loss.

Macronutrients

Your diet's main ingredients, proteins, carbs, and fats, each have a special function in the metabolism and storage of fat. You may customize your diet to support fat loss and enhance metabolic health by knowing how these macronutrients impact belly fat.

Proteins

Building and mending tissues, synthesizing hormones and enzymes, and bolstering immune system function all require proteins. Furthermore important to weight control and fat loss are they.

- ***Effects on Belly Fat***: The most filling macronutrient, protein lowers total calorie intake and prolongs feelings of fullness. This can help to sustain a calorie deficit required for fat loss and stop overeating.

- ***Effect of Thermogens***: With a high thermic impact, protein takes more energy to digest and metabolize than fats and carbs. This more energy used can help one lose weight.
- ***Preserving Muscle***: Sustaining a healthy metabolism during weight loss depends on keeping muscle mass up. Enough protein helps maintain lean muscle tissue, which promotes fat reduction and averts metabolic slowdown.
- ***Dietary Sources***: List sources include eggs, beans, lentils, and tofu as well as chicken, turkey, and fish. These selections offer little bad fat and plenty of excellent protein.
- ***Protein Supplements***: For those who need more protein or have few dietary sources, protein powders and smoothies can be easy methods to boost consumption.

Foods containing carbohydrates

Function within the Body

The main energy supply of the organism, carbohydrates power both intellectual and physical activity. But the kind and amount of carbohydrates ingested can have a big impact on how much fat builds up, particularly in the abdomen.

- ***Affect on Belly Fat***: Foods heavy in refined carbs, such pastries, sweet snacks and white bread, quickly raise blood sugar and insulin levels. Increased fat storage—especially of visceral fat—and insulin resistance may result from this.

- ***Complex Carbohydrates***: More slowly digested complex carbs found in whole grains, fruits, vegetables, and legumes lead to steadier blood sugar levels and long-lasting energy. Additionally providing fiber, these meals promote digestive health and help with satiety.
- ***Foods Low in Glycemia***: Blood sugar rises from low-glycemic index (GI) foods more gradually and slowly. Including low-GI foods like most veggies, quinoa, and oats can help control insulin levels and lower the chance of fat buildup.
- ***Foods High in Glycemia***: Consuming little high-GI meals like sugary cereals and white rice will help you avoid sharp rises in blood sugar and the ensuing fat storage.
- ***Nutritional Plans***: Give complex carbohydrates and meals high in fiber top priority when aiming for balanced carbohydrate consumption. Steer clear or cut back on added sweets and refined carbohydrates.
- ***Control of Portion***: To prevent overindulging in calories from carbohydrates—even from healthy sources—watch portion sizes. It can also help control blood sugar and improve satiety to combine carbohydrates with proteins and good fats.

Nutritional Values

Function within the Body

In order to support cell membrane integrity, supply energy, and absorb fat-soluble vitamins, diets must include fats. The kind of fat eaten is quite important in determining abdominal fat and general wellness.

- ***Impact on Belly Fat***: Processed meals, fried foods, and some animal products can all include trans and excessive saturated fats, which can increase inflammation and the buildup of visceral fat. Increased risk of metabolic problems and cardiovascular disease is associated with certain lipids.
- ***Healthy Fats***: Foods high in fatty fish, nuts, seeds and avocados include mono- and polyunsaturated fats, which are anti-inflammatory and can help lose abdominal fat. These fats balance lipid profiles and promote heart health.
- ***Dietary Sources***: Excellent sources of monounsaturated fats that can lower high cholesterol and aid in weight control are almonds, avocados, and olive oil.
- ***Polyunsaturated Fats***: Supporting metabolic health and lowering inflammation are omega-3 and omega-6 fatty acids, which are present in walnuts, flaxseeds, and fatty fish (like salmon and mackerel).
- ***The saturated fats***: Though it should be used sparingly, some saturated fat is essential. Sources are butter, coconut oil, and fatty meat cuts. Wherever you can, use leaner cuts and fats from plants.

- ***Trans Fats***: Steer clear of these whenever at all possible. Used frequently in processed and fried meals, partly hydrogenated oils include Trans fats.
- ***Nutritional Plans***: Change out the bad fats for better ones. Choose nuts and seeds over packaged treats, for instance, and use olive oil instead of butter.
- ***The Moderation***: Since even good fats are high in calories, they should be used sparingly. To keep a balanced diet, mix your fat consumption with that of proteins and carbohydrates.

Summary

Fighting abdominal fat can be effectively accomplished with nutrition. With knowledge of how nutrition contributes to fat storage and how macronutrients affect it, you may make decisions that promote both weight loss and general health. Stress a well-balanced diet low in processed foods, bad fats, refined sugars, and lean proteins but high in whole foods and complex carbs. Building on this basis, the following chapters will look at certain diet plans, workout regimens, and lifestyle modifications to help you get and stay in a leaner, healthier body.

Smart Nutritional Plans

Many times, the desire to lose belly fat drives people to investigate different eating plans. Among the most well-liked and successful are the Mediterranean, ketogenic, and low-carb diets. Every one of these methods has special advantages and may be modified to suit particular requirements   and   tastes.

Foods low in carbs

Low-carb diets emphasize proteins and lipids over carbohydrates. Because they encourage fat burning and lower insulin levels, these diets work well for weight loss and belly   fat   reduction.

- ***Insulin Regulation***: Cutting back on carbohydrates helps blood sugar levels stay steadier and lessens insulin spikes that encourage fat storage. Improved Satiety: Increased sensations of fullness brought on by a high protein and fat diet can lower total calorie consumption.
Types of Low-Carb Diets: Permits 50–150 grams of carbohydrates daily, appropriate for slow weight loss and preserving metabolic health. Strict Low-Carb: keeps carbs to less than 50 grams a day, which frequently results in faster weight loss.

  Weight Loss: Helps lose weight, especially from the abdomen.
Control of Blood Sugar: Enhances insulin sensitivity and facilitates the treatment of type 2 diabetes.
Higher consumption of fat and protein helps regulate appetite, which results in **Reduced Hunger**.

Difficulties– Adjustment Time: Fatigue and irritability are common early adverse effects when the body adjusts to consuming fewer carbohydrates. ***Nutrient Deficiency***: Chance of being deficient in vital nutrients present in foods high in carbohydrates, such as fruits and whole grains.

The Ketogenic Diet

Table of Contents

An extreme form of low-carb diet called the ketogenic (KETO) diet emphasizes a high fat intake, a moderate protein intake, and very minimal carbohydrates. A condition known as ketosis is the aim, in which the body uses fat as fuel rather than carbohydrates.

How It Works: The body enters ketosis, a metabolic state in which fat is transformed into ketones, an alternate energy source, by sharply cutting carbs to usually fewer than 20–50 grams per day.

Fat as Fuel: Eating more fat keeps one feeling full and energetic.

Rapid Weight reduction: Encourages notable fat reduction, including visceral fat.

Appetite Suppression: The inhibiting effects of fat and ketones cause one to consume fewer calories.

Mental Clarity: Ketosis has some people reporting better attention and mental clarity.

Tight Compliance Needed: To stay in ketosis, the diet requires exact macronutrient monitoring.

Exercise for Belly Fat Reduction

Physical activity is an essential component of a healthy lifestyle and has an important role in weight control and fat loss, particularly in lowering stubborn belly fat. Exercise not only burns calories, but it also improves metabolic health, boosts mood, and lowers the risk of chronic disease.

Significance of Physical Activity

- ***Cardiovascular Health***: Regular exercise strengthens the heart, improves circulation, and lowers the risk of heart disease and stroke.
- ***Metabolism Boost***: Exercise improves metabolism, allowing the body to burn more calories at rest. This is especially crucial for lowering visceral fat, which is metabolically active and associated with a variety of health concerns.
- ***Hormonal Balance***: Physical activity helps to regulate hormones like insulin and cortisol, which play important roles in fat storage and stress management.
- ***Mental Wellbeing***: Endorphins are released during exercise, which improves mood while also reducing tension, anxiety, and depression. This emotional balance can help to minimize stress-related eating, which is typically linked to belly fat.

- ***Energy Balance***: Physical exercise increases the number of calories burned, helping to create the caloric deficit required for weight loss.
- ***Fat oxidation***: Regular exercise improves the body's ability to oxidize fat for energy, which aids in the elimination of stored fat, particularly abdominal fat.

Exercises for Belly Fat Loss

The most effective way to lose belly fat is to follow a well-rounded workout program that incorporates both aerobic and strength training. Each sort of exercise provides distinct advantages that help to total fat loss and better health.

Aerobic exercises

Aerobic workouts, commonly known as cardio, are activities that raise your heart rate and respiration while repeatedly working big muscle groups. These activities are very efficient at burning calories and improving cardiovascular health.

Aerobic exercises include running and jogging. These high-impact activities are excellent for burning calories and increasing cardiovascular fitness. Running at moderate to high intensity can help you lose tummy fat.

- ***Walk***: Brisk walking is a low-impact workout that is appropriate for persons of all fitness levels. Regular walking can help you lose visceral fat and enhance your overall health.
- ***CYCLING***: Cycling, whether done outdoors or on a stationary bike, is an effective low-impact aerobic

workout that can help you burn calories and lose belly fat.

- ***Swimming***: This full-body workout is easy on the joints and extremely effective at burning calories and losing weight.
- ***Dance***: Zumba and dancing aerobics are entertaining ways to raise your heart rate and burn calories.

Benefits

- ***Caloric Burn***: Aerobic exercises burn a lot of calories, which helps create a caloric deficit and reduce belly fat.
- ***Improved Cardiovascular Health***: Regular cardio activities strengthen the heart and lungs, lowering the risk of heart disease and increasing overall cardiovascular fitness.
- ***Increased Endurance***: Aerobic exercises increase stamina and endurance, allowing you to engage in physical activities for longer periods of time.

Recommendations

- ***Frequency***: Aim for at least 150 minutes of moderate-intensity or 75 minutes of high-intensity aerobic activity per week, according to health organizations.
- ***Variation***: Use a range of aerobic activities to avoid boredom and target different muscle groups.

Strength Training

Strength training, often known as resistance training, is a set of exercises that work against resistance to build muscle strength and endurance. This can include free weights, weight machines, resistance bands, and bodyweight workouts.

Strength training includes weightlifting, which involves using free weights like dumbbells, barbells, and kettle-bells to complete movements like squats, dead-lifts, and bench presses.

- ***Bodyweight Exercises***: Push-ups, pull-ups, and planks use your own body weight as resistance.
- ***Resistance Bands***: Use elastic bands to add resistance to workouts like bicep curls and leg extensions.
- ***Machines***: Fitness equipment designed to target specific muscle regions while delivering controlled resistance.

Benefits

- ***Increased Muscle Mass***: Strength training boosts resting metabolic rate, leading to increased calorie burn.
- ***Enhanced Fat Loss***: While aerobic exercise burns calories during the activity, strength training builds muscle mass, which promotes long-term fat loss, particularly belly fat.
- ***Improved Insulin Sensitivity***: Strength training helps control blood sugar levels by increasing muscle

mass, which increases insulin sensitivity and lowers the risk of type 2 diabetes.

- ***Functional Fitness***: Increasing strength improves overall functional fitness, making daily tasks easier and lowering the chance of injury.

Recommendations

- ***Frequency***: Perform strength training exercises at least 2-3 times each week, addressing all main muscle groups.
- ***Progressive Overload***: Gradually increase the weight or resistance used in strength training exercises to keep your muscles challenged and growing.

Integrating Aerobic and Strength Training

Combining aerobic workouts and strength training offers a holistic approach to losing belly fat and enhancing general fitness. Here's how you can successfully incorporate both types of workout into your routine:

- ***Weekly Schedule***: Create a weekly fitness plan that incorporates both aerobic and strength training activities. To achieve balanced fitness growth, alternate between cardio and strength training days.
- ***Circuit Training***: Circuit training allows you to combine aerobic and strength workouts into one workout session. This is executing a series of exercises

in quick succession with little rest, effectively burning calories while increasing muscle.

- ***High Intensity Interval Training (HIIT):*** HIIT workouts consist of short bursts of intense activity followed by intervals of relaxation or lower-intensity exercise. HIIT can combine both aerobic and strength training, making it an efficient approach to burn fat and build muscle.
- ***Integrate Lifestyle***: Incorporate more physical exercise into your regular routine by walking or cycling to work, taking the stairs, or participating in leisure sports.
- ***Consistency***: Consistency is essential. Create a regular fitness plan that matches your lifestyle and stick to it for long-term effects.

Conclusion

Exercise is an effective way to reduce belly fat and improve overall health. A combination of aerobic workouts and strength training is the most efficient way to achieve and maintain a leaner body. Aerobic workouts burn calories and promote cardiovascular health, but strength training increases muscle growth and metabolism. By incorporating both types of exercise into a balanced routine and making physical activity a regular part of your life, you may efficiently reduce belly fat and improve your overall health. In the next chapters, we will look at further lifestyle modifications and psychological tactics to help you on your journey to a healthier, fitter body.

Exercise and Abdominal Fat Reduction

High-Intensity Interval Training (HIIT) is a very successful workout approach that involves short bursts of intense activity followed by intervals of lower-intensity exercise or rest. This type of workout increases calorie burn, improves cardiovascular fitness, and speeds up fat reduction, making it very useful for decreasing belly fat.

High Intensity Interval Training (HIIT)

How HIIT Works

- ***Intensity Bursts***: High-intensity intervals push your body to its limits, increasing heart rate and calorie burn.
- ***Recovery Periods***: The lower-intensity intervals allow for partial recovery, allowing you to exert maximum effort during the intense bursts.
- ***EPOC Effect***: HIIT causes excess post-exercise oxygen consumption (EPOC), which means that your body continues to burn calories at a higher rate even after the workout is over.

Benefits of HIIT

- ***Time Efficiency***: HIIT workouts can be done in less time than regular cardio, making them suitable for hectic schedules.
- ***Enhanced Fat Loss***: HIIT is particularly effective in reducing visceral fat, which collects around the abdomen.

- ***Improved Cardiovascular Health***: HIIT boosts heart health and VO2 max (the amount of oxygen your body can use during exercise).
- ***Muscle Retention***: High-intensity interval training can help you retain and even develop muscle mass while losing weight.

Examples of HIIT Workouts

- ***Tabatha***: This protocol contains 20 seconds of maximal effort followed by 10 seconds of rest, repeated 8 times (4 minutes total).
- ***Sprint Intervals***: Sprint for 30 seconds, then walk or jog for 1-2 minutes.
- ***Circuit Training***: Performing activities such as burpees, jumping jacks, and mountain climbers in a circuit pattern with little rest in between.
- ***Bodyweight HIIT***: Exercises including push-ups, squats, and lunges are done at a high intensity with brief rest intervals.

Tips for Effective HIIT

- ***Warm-Up***: Begin with a warm-up to prepare muscles and avoid damage.
- ***Good Form***: Maintain good form, even during high-intensity intervals, to prevent injury.
- ***Gradual Progression***: Begin with shorter intervals, gradually increasing the intensity and length as your fitness increases.

- **Recovery**: Allow enough time for recovery between HIIT workouts to avoid overtraining and encourage muscle healing.

Developing an Effective Workout Plan

An efficient training regimen should be adjusted to your specific fitness level, goals, and tastes. A good plan relies on consistency, variation, and advancement.

Personalized Approach

Assessing Fitness Level

- **Initial Assessment**: Test your current fitness level with timed runs, push-ups, and flexibility assessments.
- **Setting Goals**: Define specific, measurable goals, such as decreasing belly fat, increasing cardiovascular endurance, or growing muscle.

Elements of an Effective Workout Plan

- **Cardiovascular Training**: Include aerobic workouts like jogging, cycling, and swimming to boost heart health and burn calories.
- **Strength Training**: Perform workouts that target all main muscle groups at least twice or three times each week.
- **Flexibility and Mobility**: Stretching and mobility exercises can help you increase your flexibility, avoid injuries, and perform better overall.

- ***Rest and Recovery***: Plan rest days to allow your body to heal and repair, so avoiding overtraining and injury.

Weekly Workout Schedule

Beginners Example Plan

- ***Monday***: 30 minutes of brisk walking or light jogging followed by 15 minutes of bodyweight strength training (squats, push-ups, and planks).
- ***Tuesday***: HIIT workout (20 minutes) with bodyweight exercises.
- ***Wednesday***: Rest or gentle exercise (yoga, stretching).
- ***Thursday***: 30 minutes of cycling or swimming and 15 minutes of core workouts (crunches, leg lifts).
- ***Friday***: Full-body strength workout (with dumbbells or resistance bands).
- ***Saturday:*** HIIT workout (20 minutes) with aerobic and strength exercises.
- ***Sunday***: Rest or light activities (such as walking or stretching).

Intermediate/Advanced Example Plan

- ***Monday***: 45 minutes of high-intensity cycling or jogging, followed by upper-body strength training.
- ***Tuesday***: HIIT training (30 minutes) including sprint intervals.
- ***Wednesday***: Active recuperation (mild yoga, walking) and flexibility training.

- ***Thursday***: Full-body strength exercise using free weights and machines.
- ***Friday***: 30 minutes of swimming or rowing plus a core workout.
- ***Saturday***: HIIT workout (30 minutes) focusing on explosive movements (e.g., jump squats, burpees).
- ***Sunday***: Rest or light activities (such as hiking or stretching).

Progression and Adaptation

- ***Gradual Increase***: Challenge your body by gradually increasing the intensity, duration, and complexity of your workouts.
- ***Listen to Your Body***: Be aware of indicators of weariness and alter your workout intensity and rest intervals accordingly.
- ***Regular Assessment***: To ensure continuous growth, examine your fitness level and goals on a regular basis and change your workout schedule accordingly.

Common Exercise Myths

Myth 1

- ***Spot Reduction Is Reality***: Targeting a specific location for fat loss through exercise is a fallacy. Fat loss happens throughout the body due to a calorie shortage and hereditary variables.
- ***Solution***: A balanced diet and full-body workouts will help you lose overall body fat, including belly fat.

Myth 2

- ***More Exercise = Better Results***: Regular exercise is beneficial, but more is not necessarily better. Overtraining can cause injury, burnout, and poor outcomes.
- ***Solution***: Incorporate rest and recovery days into your exercise routine. Quality and consistency in workouts are more important than quantity.

Myth 3

- ***Cardio is the Only Way to Lose Belly Fat***: Strength training is essential for building muscle and improving metabolism, in addition to cardio for calorie burning.
- ***Solution***: To maximize fat reduction and muscle development, combine cardiovascular and strength training routines.

Myth 4

- ***Crunches and Sit-Ups are the Best Exercises for Belly Fat***: While crunches and sit-ups can develop abdominal muscles, they do not directly target belly fat.
- ***Solution***: Use a mix of workouts, such as aerobic, weight training, and core exercises, to efficiently reduce belly fat and strengthen your core.

Myth 5

- ***Weightlifting Makes Women Bulky***: Weightlifting does not typically result in bulky muscles for women due to hormonal differences. Strength exercise helps to build lean muscle, improve tone, and increase metabolism.
- ***Solution***: Women should incorporate strength training into their workout routines to improve muscular tone, strength, and general fitness.

Summary

Exercise is an essential part of losing abdominal fat and increasing overall health. High-Intensity Interval Training (HIIT) is a quick and efficient approach to burn calories and reduce visceral fat. Developing an effective workout regimen that incorporates a mix of cardiovascular, strength, and flexibility workouts is critical for long-term improvement. Avoiding common workout myths and understanding the reality of fat reduction will allow you to make more educated decisions and optimize your fitness journey. In the following chapters, we'll look at other lifestyle modifications and psychological tactics to supplement your exercise and nutrition efforts, assuring a comprehensive approach to obtaining and maintaining a leaner, healthier physique.

Belly Fat and Lifestyle Factors

Often disregarded yet just as important for fat loss and general wellness is sleep. Enough sleep is necessary for energy balance, hormone control, and healing—all of which affect body weight and fat distribution.

Sleep and Its Effect on Fat Loss

- ***Hormonal Balance***: Sleep controls important hormones linked to appetite and satiety, such as leptin and ghrelin. The hunger hormone ghrelin rises with sleep deprivation and so does appetite. As leptin, which indicates fullness, drops, and overeating results?

- ***Insulin Sensitivity***: The body finds it more difficult to properly handle glucose when insulin sensitivity is reduced by poor sleep. Higher blood sugar and more fat storing, especially in the abdomen, may result from this.

- ***Cortisol Levels***: Stress hormone cortisol is increased when one is sleep deprived. Especially visceral fat around the abdomen, increased cortisol levels encourage fat buildup.

Effects of Sleep Deprivation

- **Increased desires**: Weight gain is typically exacerbated by desires for foods high in calories and carbohydrates.
- **Lower Physical Activity**: Lack of sleep can sap motivation and energy, which lowers calorie expenditure and physical activity.
- **Metabolic Slowdown**: Reduced resting metabolic rate caused by chronic sleep loss can impede the effective burning of calories.

Tips for Getting More Sleep

- **Regular Sleep Schedule**: Set aside time each day to go to bed and wake up, including on the weekends.
- **Sleep Environment**: Maintaining the bedroom calm, cool, and dark will help you sleep well. When in doubt, use white noise machines, earplugs, or blackout curtains.
- **Sleep Hygiene**: Make a soothing bedtime ritual out of reading, meditation, or a warm bath. At least one hour before bed, stay away from screens and other electronics because the blue light can interfere with the synthesis of melatonin.
- **Restricted Stimulants**: Take no coffee or nicotine in the late afternoon or evening. Moderate drinking is also advised because it can interfere with sleep.

Handling Stress

A big contributing element to weight increase and fat distribution—especially belly fat—is stress. Hormone reactions brought on by chronic stress boost hunger and encourage fat storage.

The Science of Stress and Fat Storage

- **Cortisol**: Cortisol levels rise with ongoing stress. An appetite and a desire for fatty and sugary foods are increased by high cortisol levels, which can lead to weight gain. The more metabolically active and associated with health hazards visceral fat is also encouraged to be stored by cortisol.
- **Behavioral Inputs**: Stress frequently results in emotional eating, when people eat comfort foods heavy in fat, sugar, and calories. This kind of behavior makes fat storage and weight increase worse.

Stress Management Strategies That Work

- **Meditation and Mindfulness**: Through their promotion of relaxation and mental clarity, mindfulness and meditation practices can help lower stress. Methods that work include guided imagery, progressive muscle relaxation, and deep breathing.
- **Physical Exercise**: Stress can be effectively managed by regular exercise. Exercise lowers cortisol, produces endorphins, the body's natural mood enhancers, and enhances mental health generally.

- ***Healthy Relationships***: Stress can be lowered and emotional support can be obtained by developing and preserving encouraging relationships. Engaging in group activities, chatting to friends or family, and socializing can all help one become more resilient emotionally. To efficiently manage time, arrange and rank chores. Realistic goals broken down into doable steps can lower stress and increase output.
- ***Passions & Interests***: Taking part in enjoyable pursuits and pastimes might help you relax and raise your level of life satisfaction generally.

Alcohol Use

Fat buildup can be greatly impacted by alcohol use, especially in the abdomen. Fat loss that works requires an understanding of the connection between alcohol and weight gain.

The Science of Alcoholism and Fat Storage

- ***Caloric Content***: When weighed against proteins and carbs, alcohol has a comparatively high seven calories per gram. These worthless calories do nothing for your health other than add to weight increase.
- ***Protein***: The liver gives alcohol, when ingested, priority for metabolism over other nutrients. Fat accumulation is promoted by this slowing down the metabolism of fats and carbs.
- ***Controlling Your Hunger and Impulses***: Drinking alcohol might make one more hungry and

less inhibited, which can result in overeating and bad meal selections. We call this eating high-calorie, unhealthy foods "drunken munchies."

Alcohol's Effects on Belly Fat

- ***Visceral Fat***: Alcohol encourages the buildup of this dangerous kind of fat that envelops internal organs and raises the chance of metabolic disorders.
- ***Hormonal Disturbance***: Alcohol can upset the balance of hormones, including cortisol and insulin, which are involved in the distribution and storage of fat.

Alcohol Consumption Management Strategies

- ***Moderation***: Keep alcohol intake to reasonable levels, which are one drink for women and two drinks for men per day.
- ***Better Selections***: Steer clear of sweet mixers and go for lower-calorie alcoholic drinks like wine or light beer. To stay hydrated and cut back total consumption, sip water in between alcoholic beverages.
- ***Concentrated Drinking***: Watch when you drink and make an effort to cut less on alcohol while you're losing weight. Set yourself limits and make plans in advance to prevent overindulging.
- ***Days without Drinking***: Add days without alcohol to your week to cut back on your total consumption and allow your body to heal.

Smoking and Its Consequence

In brief

Among the many negative health consequences of smoking are changes to weight and fat distribution. Because smoking suppresses appetite, it is sometimes linked to weight loss; in reality, smoking adds to unhealthy fat distribution, especially belly fat.

The Science of Smoking and Fat Distribution

- *Nicotine and Metabolism*: One stimulant in cigarettes called nicotine can speed up metabolism and lessen appetite. Still, the negative consequences on health and fat distribution exceed the advantages of weight management.
- *Insulin Resistance*: Smoking makes one more resistant to insulin, which raises blood sugar and encourages the storage of fat—especially visceral fat.
- *Inflammation*: Inflammation and oxidative stress brought on by smoking raise the risk of metabolic disorders and help the body store belly fat.

Belly fat effects of smoking

- *Accumulation of visceral fat:* Generally speaking, smokers have more visceral fat than non-smokers. Because it surrounds internal organs and is associated with major health problems, this kind of fat is very harmful.

- ***The Altered Hormonal Balance***: Insulin and cortisol, hormones involved in the distribution and storage of fat, are impacted by smoking. Smoking-related raised cortisol can cause belly fat to grow.
- ***Behavioral Therapy***: Counseling and behavioral therapy can assist address the psychological components of nicotine addiction and offer quitting techniques.
- ***Nicotine Replacement Therapy***: Cravings and withdrawal symptoms can be lessened with the use of nicotine patches, gum, and lozenges.
- ***Medications***: By lessening cravings and withdraw symptoms, prescription drugs like varenicline and bupropion can help people stop smoking.
- ***Support Groups***: Enrolling in programs like as Nicotine Anonymous or support groups might offer encouragement and assistance from other people who are also giving up.
- ***Healthy Substitutes***: Take up exercise, hobbies, or stress-reduction strategies as options to smoking.

Summary

Fat buildup is mostly caused by lifestyle choices including smoking, drinking, stress management, and sleep. Hormonal balance and avoiding weight gain need enough sleep and good stress management. Limiting abdominal fat and enhancing general health need limiting alcohol intake and giving up smoking. You may improve your attempts at getting a leaner, healthier body by taking care of these lifestyle elements. We shall look at holistic methods and psychological techniques in the upcoming chapters to help you on your path to the best possible health and well-being.

PHASE FIVE

Belly Fat and Supplements

Review of Supplements for Burning Fat

Widely promoted as easy fixes for losing belly fat and getting a leaner body are fat-burning pills. These pills make the claims to boost energy expenditure, speed up metabolism, and encourage fat oxidation. It's important to realize, nevertheless, that whilst certain supplements can be beneficial, others might not have any scientific backing or might even be harmful to health.

Categories of Supplements for Burning Fat

- Thermals: Components in these supplements are supposed to boost thermo-genesis, the body's process of producing heat and burning calories. Caffeine, extract from green tea, and capsaicin are common components.

- *Anti-Appetite Drugs*: These pills say they will help you eat fewer calories by reducing hunger and cravings. Many times, this is achieved using ingredients like fiber, glucomannan, and 5-HTP.

- *The Metabolism Boosters*: By raising metabolic rate, these supplements hope to enhance calorie burning. Complements that increase metabolism often include L-carnitine, conjugated linoleic acid (CLA), and forskolin.

- **_The Fat Blockers_**: These supplements supposedly stop the body from storing dietary fats by blocking their absorption. Among the substances that block fat are chitosan, white kidney bean extract, and orlistat.

Knowing Supplement Regulation

It is noteworthy that national laws governing dietary supplements differ, and many supplements are not subject to the same stringent testing and supervision as prescription medications. The effectiveness and safety of fat-burning supplements may therefore not have been sufficiently proven.

Side Effects and Risks

When taken exactly as suggested, some fat-burning supplements might be generally regarded as safe, but others could have some hazards and adverse consequences. Among these are heightened heart rate, high blood pressure, stomach problems, sleeplessness, and in severe cases, liver damage. Before beginning any new supplement program, especially if you are using medication or have a history of medical issues, it is imperative that you speak with a healthcare provider.

Supplements Supported by Evidence

A First Look at Supplements Based on Evidence

Even while there is no shortage of fat-burning products on the market with wild promises, it is important to concentrate on those that have solid scientific backing. Clinical research has shown that evidence-based supplements can help with fat loss and metabolic health improvement.

To be sure fat-burning supplements are safe and supported by evidence, take into account the following:

- ***Clinical Research***: Search for supplements that have been investigated in properly planned clinical trials including human subjects. Examine the study design, sample size, time frame, and quantified results.
- ***Transparency and Credibility***: Select supplements from reliable producers who disclose openly details about the contents, suppliers, and production methods. Seek for accreditations from reputable outside sources like ConsumerLab.com or NSF International.
- ***Safety Profile***: Evaluate the supplement's possible adverse effects and interactions with other drugs or supplements. Should you have any worries or underlying medical issues, speak with a medical practitioner.
- ***Dose and Formulation***: Take into account the supplement's formulation and dose as well as the

bioavailability of its active components. Seek for supplements that use premium formulations for best absorption and deliver clinically appropriate amounts of important components.

- ***Realistic Expectations***: Recognize that supplements are not weight reduction miracle cures and control your expectations. They have to be a component of a whole plan that also involves a balanced diet, consistent exercise, and lifestyle changes.

Supplements Based on Research for Fat Loss

Although everyone reacts differently to supplements, scientific studies have indicated that a number of components may help with fat loss and metabolic health. Among supplements supported by research are:

- ***The stimulant caffeine***: It promotes fat oxidation, and enhances exercise performance. It has been researched for possible advantages in weight control and is often included in fat-burning supplements.
- ***Green Tea Extract***: Compounds called catechins have been demonstrated to increase metabolism and encourage the oxidation of fat. Research indicates that, especially in conjunction with exercise, taking green tea extract supplements may help with fat loss.
- ***Yohimbine:*** The yohimbe tree's bark yields an alkaloid called yohimbine, which has been investigated for possible fat-loss benefits. Its mechanisms of action are raising adrenaline levels

and encouraging the release of fatty acids from fat cells so that they may be used as energy.

- ***Conjugated Linoleic Acid (CLA):*** CLA is a class of fatty acid present in dairy and meat products as well as in supplements. Though the data are conflicting, research indicates that using CLA supplements may help lower body fat mass, especially abdominal fat.

- ***Forskolin***: Researched for its possible impact on fat metabolism, forskolin is an extract from the roots of the Coleus forskohlii plant. According to some research, taking forskolin supplements may assist reduce waist circumference and body fat percentage.

About

Although fat-burning pills are routinely promoted as easy fixes for lowering belly fat, one should approach them cautiously and skeptically. While certain supplements might be beneficial, others might not have any scientific backing or might even be harmful to health. When looking at fat-burning supplements, go for those that have been clinically tested and shown real advantages in assisting in fat loss and enhancing metabolic health. Prioritize also lifestyle elements like nutrition, exercise, sleep, and stress management because these are essential to reaching and keeping a healthy weight and body composition. Before beginning any new supplement program, always speak with a healthcare provider, particularly if you are taking medication or have a history of medical issues.

Evidence-Based Supplements for Fat Loss

Evidence-based supplements can help you lose weight and get a leaner body when combined with a healthy diet and regular exercise. Let's look at three substances that have received attention for their ability to aid in fat loss:

Green Tea Extract

Green tea extract is made from the leaves of the Camellia sinensis plant and has been eaten for millennia for its numerous health benefits. It includes beneficial chemicals known as catechins, the most prevalent and extensively studied of which is epigallocatechin gallate (EGCG).

Mechanism of Action

- **Thermo-genesis**: EGCG has been found to boost thermo-genesis, the body's process of producing heat and burning calories. This impact is assumed to be mediated by the activation of brown adipose tissue, which regulates energy consumption.
- **Fat Oxidation**: Green tea extract may help the body use stored fat for energy more efficiently. This can help with general fat loss, especially abdominal fat.
- **Metabolic Rate**: According to certain research, green tea extract intake can boost metabolic rate, resulting in higher calorie expenditure even at rest.

Research Evidence

- ***Weight loss***: Several clinical investigations have shown that green tea extract intake can result in mild weight loss and reduced body fat percentage. These effects tend to be stronger when paired with calorie restriction and exercise.
- ***Abdominal fat:*** Evidence suggests that green tea extract may reduce visceral fat, which accumulates around organs and is linked to metabolic health problems.
- ***Optimal Dosage and Standardized Extracts***: Look for green tea extract pills that are standardized to contain a certain percentage of EGCG, usually between 50% and 95%. The most typical EGCG dosages utilized in trials ranged from 250 mg to 500 mg per day.
- ***Time***: Green tea extract can be consumed with or between meals, depending on personal preference and tolerance. It is generally well accepted, though some people may experience minor stomach discomfort.

Caffeine

Caffeine is a naturally occurring stimulant present in many foods and beverages, including coffee, tea, and chocolate. It is well-known for increasing alertness and energy, but it may also help with fat loss and workout performance.

Mechanism of Action

- ***Metabolic Rate***: Caffeine stimulates the central nervous system, resulting in higher metabolic rate and calorie expenditure. This impact can boost fat burning and aid in weight loss, especially when accompanied with physical activity.
- ***Fat oxidation***: Caffeine has been demonstrated to boost fatty acid oxidation, making them more readily available for energy usage. This can conserve muscle glycogen during exercise and increase endurance.
- ***Appetite Suppression***: According to some study, caffeine may suppress appetite and reduce energy intake, albeit the mechanisms are not entirely understood.

Research Evidence

- ***Fat Loss***: Numerous researches have looked into the benefits of coffee on fat loss and weight management. Caffeine supplementation has been demonstrated to produce small decreases in body weight and fat mass, with higher effects observed in caffeine-naive people or during short-term use.
- ***Exercise performance***: Caffeine administration has been linked to increased endurance, strength, and power output during exercise. These performance increases can increase calorie expenditure and fat reduction over time.

- ***Optimal Dosage and Individual Tolerance***: Caffeine sensitivity varies by each, so start with a modest dose and gradually increase as tolerated. The recommended dosage for fat loss is commonly 100 mg to 400 mg per day, divided into many doses as needed.
- ***Time***: Caffeine can be used before exercise to improve performance and fat loss. Before avoid sleep problems, avoid ingesting caffeine close before bedtime.

Conjugated Linoleic Acid (CLA)

Conjugated linoleic acid (CLA) is a type of fatty acid found naturally in meat and dairy products, particularly those derived from grass-fed animals. It has received attention for its possible impact on body composition and fat loss.

Mechanism of Action

- ***Fat Metabolism***: CLA is thought to improve fat metabolism by enhancing the activity of enzymes involved in fatty acid oxidation. This can lead to a greater use of stored fat for energy, resulting in fat loss.
- ***Lean body mass***: Some evidence suggests that CLA supplementation may help preserve lean body mass during calorie restriction, reducing muscle mass loss that is commonly associated with weight loss.

Research Evidence

- ***Body Composition***: Clinical research looking into the impact of CLA supplementation on body composition has yielded varied results. While some research indicated decreases in body fat percentage and waist circumference, others found no meaningful effects.
- ***Metabolic health***: There is modest evidence that CLA supplementation may improve insulin sensitivity, blood lipid profiles, and inflammation, all of which are crucial for metabolic health.

Optimal Dosage

- ***Supplement Format***: CLA supplements come in a variety of formats, including softgels, capsules, and powder. Look for CLA supplements that include a standardized dose of 1,000 mg to 3,000 mg per day.
- ***Duration***: It may take several weeks or months of consistent supplementation to see significant changes in body composition. For optimal effects, combine CLA supplementation with a well-balanced diet and regular exercise.

Possible Side Effects and Risks

Green tea extract, caffeine, and CLA are usually regarded safe when used as intended, however they may cause negative effects in some people. It is critical to be aware of these potential hazards and check with a healthcare practitioner before beginning any new supplement regimen, especially if you have underlying health concerns or are using drugs.

- ***Caffeine Sensitivity***: Caffeine in green tea extract might induce jitteriness, anxiety, sleeplessness, and elevated heart rate in sensitive persons.
- ***Gastrointestinal distress***: Some people may have digestive problems such as nausea, stomach distress, or diarrhea after taking green tea extract supplements, especially on an empty stomach.
- ***Toxicity to the Liver:*** While rare, there have been reports of liver damage from high-dose green tea extract use. It is critical to adhere to authorized dosages and watch for any signs of liver dysfunction.
- ***Insomnia***: Caffeine, a central nervous system stimulant, can disrupt sleep, especially when eaten in high amounts or late in the day.
- ***Anxiety and jitters***: Excessive caffeine consumption can cause anxiety, uneasiness, restlessness, and jitteriness, particularly in caffeine-sensitive persons.
- ***Heart palpitations***: Caffeine in high dosages can produce palpitations, rapid heart rate, and high blood pressure, particularly in people with pre-existing cardiovascular disorders.

Conjugated Linoleic Acid (CLA)

- ***Digestive Issues***: Taking greater doses of CLA supplements may cause abdominal discomfort, bloating, or diarrhea.
- ***Insulin Sensitivity***: There is some concern that long-term CLA supplementation may compromise insulin sensitivity in certain people, although additional research is needed to validate this possibility.
- ***Blood Lipids***: CLA supplementation has been linked with changes in blood lipid levels, including increases in

Medical and Surgical Interventions

In some circumstances, lifestyle changes and dietary supplements may not be enough to produce significant fat loss, especially for people with stubborn belly fat. Medical and surgical therapies provide additional alternatives for those looking for more aggressive ways to reduce unwanted fat deposits. This chapter delves into numerous approaches, including when to seek medical attention, prescription drugs, and non-surgical procedures like Cool Sculpting.

Assessment and evaluation

Before considering medical procedures for fat loss, a healthcare expert should conduct a thorough assessment and evaluation. This may involve:

Seeking Medical Help

- ***Medical History***: Go over your medical history, including any underlying health concerns, medications, and past weight loss attempts.
- ***Physical Examination***: A physical examination is performed to evaluate overall health, body composition, and fat distribution.
- ***Diagnostic Tests***: Obtaining diagnostic tests such as blood tests, imaging investigations (e.g.,

ultrasound, MRI), and metabolic assessments to check metabolic health and identify potential causes of weight increase.

Indications for Medical Care

Medical therapies for fat loss can be considered in the following situations:

- ***Obesity:*** People with a body mass index (BMI) of 30 or greater may benefit from medical therapies, particularly if they have obesity-related health issues including diabetes, hypertension, or sleep apnea.
- ***Abdominal Obesity***: People with excess abdominal fat, particularly visceral fat, may benefit from focused therapies to lower the health risks associated with central obesity.
- ***Failure of Lifestyle Modifications***: People who have tried and failed to lose significant weight by diet, exercise, and other lifestyle changes should seek medical attention for additional assistance.
- ***Health concerns***: The presence of obesity-related health concerns such as insulin resistance, dyslipidemia, or cardiovascular disease may necessitate medical intervention to avoid future consequences.

Prescription Medications

Prescription weight loss drugs are normally reserved for people who are obese or overweight and have serious health hazards. These drugs act by suppressing appetite, lowering calorie intake, or modifying fat absorption, which results in weight loss over time.

Several prescription drugs have been approved by regulatory agencies, including the United States Food and Drug Administration (FDA), for the treatment of obesity and weight management. This includes:

Common Prescription Medication

- **Phentermine**: Phentermine is a stimulant that reduces appetite and improves weight loss by raising norepinephrine levels in the brain. Because of its propensity for abuse and dependence, it is normally only recommended for brief periods of time.
- **Orlistat**: Orlistat is a lipase inhibitor that prevents the absorption of dietary fats in the intestines, resulting in lower calorie intake and weight loss. It comes in both prescription and over-the-counter (OTC) versions.
- **Liraglutide**: Liraglutide is a GLP-1 receptor agonist that was originally licensed to treat type 2 diabetes. It has also been approved for weight management in higher doses, where it reduces hunger and increases feelings of fullness.

- ***Considerations and Side Effects***: Prescription weight loss drugs may have the following potential adverse effects and considerations:
- ***Adverse effects***: Common side effects of weight reduction drugs include nausea, diarrhea, constipation, dry mouth, and sleeplessness. Some drugs may also raise heart rate or blood pressure.
- ***Safety profile***: It is critical to evaluate the safety profile of prescription drugs with a healthcare professional, including any potential interactions with other medications and underlying health issues.
- ***Monitoring***: Regular monitoring by a healthcare provider is required while taking prescription weight reduction drugs to examine efficacy, safety, and any side effects.

Non-Surgical Procedures

Nonsurgical fat removal methods provide minimally invasive alternatives to traditional surgical liposuction. These procedures often target specific areas of fat buildup and may be appropriate for people who have stubborn belly fat that doesn't respond to diet or exercise.

Cool Sculpting

Cool Sculpting, also known as cryolipolysis, is a non-invasive fat reduction process that involves freezing and eliminating fat cells beneath the skin. The treatment targets and freezes fat cells while sparing surrounding tissues, resulting in gradual fat reduction over several weeks to months.

During a Cool Sculpting session, a specialized applicator is put on a specific part of the body, such as the belly, and regulated chilling is used to freeze fat cells. Over time, the frozen fat cells die (apoptosis) and are normally removed from the body via the lymphatic system.

Benefits

Cool Sculpting has various advantages for fat reduction, including:

- ***Non-Invasive***: Cool Sculpting requires no surgery, incisions, or anesthesia, making it a low-risk procedure with little downtime.
- ***Localized Fat Reduction***: Cool Sculpting targets specific areas of fat buildup, enabling precise body contouring and shaping.
- ***Gradual Results***: Cool Sculpting produces gradual and natural-looking fat removal that occurs over several weeks to months after treatment.
- ***Minimum Discomfort***: During the procedure, patients may feel cold, numb, or tingly for a short time, although the discomfort is usually minimal.

Considerations and Side Effects

While Cool Sculpting is deemed safe and successful for the majority of people, the following concerns and potential adverse effects should be taken into account:

- ***Skin Sensations***: Temporary sensations of cold, numbness, or tingling may occur during and after the operation, although they usually recover on their own after a few weeks.
- ***Bruising and Swelling***: Some patients may develop minor bruising, swelling, or redness at the treatment site, which typically resolves within a few days.
- ***Rare Complications***: Rare complications, such as paradoxical adipose hyperplasia (PAH), in which fat cells grow rather than shrink, can occur but are uncommon.

Patient selection

Cool Sculpting is best suited for those who are near to their desired body weight but have stubborn fat pockets that refuse to go away with diet or exercise. It is not a weight-loss solution for obesity or a replacement for a healthy lifestyle.

Conclusion

Medical and surgical therapies provide additional choices for people who want to lose persistent belly fat but are unable to do so through typical lifestyle changes. Prescription drugs may be considered for patients with obesity or substantial health hazards, and non-surgical techniques like as Cool Sculpting offer less intrusive alternatives to surgical liposuction. Before choosing medical interventions, it is critical to get a thorough evaluation by a healthcare professional who can evaluate potential risks, benefits, and options. Ultimately, the solution should be personalized to the individual's needs, preferences, and overall health goals.

Ultrasound Fat Reduction

Ultrasound fat reduction, also known as ultrasound cavitations or non-invasive body contouring, is a popular cosmetic procedure that reduces localized fat without surgery. This procedure uses focused ultrasonic energy to target and destroy fat cells beneath the skin, resulting in their progressive disintegration and evacuation from the body.

The Mechanism of Action

During an ultrasonic fat reduction operation, a handheld device is utilized to provide focused ultrasound waves to the treated area, such as the belly or thighs. The ultrasonic radiation passes through the skin and heats the fat cells to a particular temperature, causing them to burst and discharge their contents into the surrounding tissue.

Procedure

The ultrasonic energy targets fat cells only, leaving surrounding tissues such as skin, muscle, and nerves untouched. To attain the best outcomes, the operation is usually conducted in many sessions separated by several weeks. During the process, patients may feel mild discomfort or a warm sensation, although this is usually tolerable.

Benefits

Ultrasound fat reduction has various advantages for people looking for non-surgical fat loss methods, including:

- ***Non-Invasive***: Ultrasound fat reduction requires no incisions, anesthesia, or downtime, making it a safe and easy alternative for many patients.
- ***Localized Fat Reduction***: The technique can target specific areas of fat buildup, allowing for more accurate body sculpting and shaping.
- ***Gradual Results***: Ultrasound fat reduction produces gradual and natural-looking fat loss over several weeks to months after treatment.
- ***Minimal Side Effects***: Most patients suffer only minor side effects, such as moderate redness, swelling, or bruising at the treatment site, which usually fades on its own within a few days.

Considerations and limitations

While ultrasonic fat reduction is usually regarded as safe and effective, it may not be appropriate for everyone. Factors to consider are:

- ***Patient Selection***: Ultrasound fat reduction is best suited for people who are near to their optimal body weight but have persistent fat deposits that resist diet and exercise.
- ***Skin Tightening***: While ultrasonic waves can help break down fat cells, it may not have a major skin

tightening effect. Additional treatments may be required to treat skin laxity or sagging.

- ***The Results***: Ultrasound fat removal results may vary depending on individual factors such as skin elasticity, fat distribution, and lifestyle behaviors. Multiple sessions may be required to attain the desired outcome.

Surgical Options for Fat Reduction

Liposuction.

Liposuction is a surgical treatment used to remove excess fat from certain parts of the body, such as the belly, thighs, hips, buttocks, and arms. It is one of the most popular cosmetic treatments in the world, with the potential to significantly change body contour and shape.

Liposuction involves making small incisions in the skin and inserting a thin tube known as a cannula into the targeted fat deposits. The cannula is attached to a vacuum device or suction pump, which removes extra fat cells and shapes the appropriate contours.

Types of Liposuction

- ***Traditional Liposuction***: This treatment includes manually removing fat cells with a suction instrument while under general or local anesthesia and sedation.

- ***Tumescent Liposuction***: Tumescent liposuction involves injecting a solution containing saline, local anesthetic, and epinephrine into the treatment area to numb it, constrict blood vessels, and enable fat removal.
- ***Laser-Assisted Liposuction***: Laser liposuction uses laser energy to liquefy fat cells before suctioning them out, resulting in less harm to surrounding tissues and perhaps shorter recovery times.

Benefits

Liposuction has various advantages for people looking for surgical fat reduction solutions, including:

- ***Dramatic Results***: Liposuction can significantly improve body contour and shape, especially in areas with resistant fat deposits.
- ***Customization***: The process can be tailored to specific areas of concern, allowing for precise sculpting and reshaping of the body.
- ***Long-term Fat Loss***: Liposuction permanently removes fat cells from the body, resulting in long-term results when properly maintained through diet and exercise.

Considerations and risks

While liposuction is generally safe when performed by a trained and experienced plastic surgeon, it is important to consider potential risks and problems such as:

- ***Bruising and Swelling***: Following liposuction, bruising, swelling, and soreness are normal side effects that usually diminish within a few weeks.
- ***Imperfections***: In some circumstances, liposuction may produce uneven shapes, skin imperfections, or asymmetry, necessitating additional touch-up procedures.
- ***Skin laxity***: Liposuction eliminates excess fat, however it may not treat loose or sagging skin. Additional surgeries, such as a belly tuck (abdominoplasty), may be required to tighten and firm the skin.

Abdominoplasty

Abdominoplasty, sometimes known as a tummy tuck, is a surgical operation that removes extra skin and fat from the abdomen while tightening the underlying muscles, yielding a flatter, more toned abdominal contour. It is frequently used in conjunction with liposuction to accomplish total abdominal rejuvenation.

An abdominoplasty surgery involves making an incision down the lower abdomen, usually below the bikini line, to reach the underlying tissues. Excess skin and fat are removed, and the abdominal muscles are tightened and mended with sutures to form a tighter abdominal wall. The leftover skin is then redraped and sutured into place, creating a smoother, more contoured abdomen.

Types of Abdominoplasty

- ***Traditional abdominoplasty***: This method is appropriate for people with moderate to severe skin laxity and abdominal fat deposits. It calls for a longer incision along the lower abdomen, as well as more thorough tissue excision and muscle tightness.
- ***Mini Abdominoplasty***: Mini abdominoplasty is best suited for people with mild to moderate skin laxity and localized fat deposits below the navel. It has a smaller incision and requires less tissue removal, making it a less invasive procedure with faster recovery times.

Benefits

Abdominoplasty has various advantages for people who want to remove excess abdominal skin and fat, including:

- ***Improved Abdominal Contour***: Abdominoplasty can significantly enhance abdominal contour, resulting in a flatter, more toned appearance.
- ***Muscle Repair***: The procedure can repair and tighten damaged or divided abdominal muscles (diastasis recti), hence restoring core strength and stability.
- ***Increased self-confidence***: A firmer, more contoured abdomen can increase self-esteem and

body confidence, making people feel more comfortable and confident about their look.

Considerations and risks

While abdominoplasty can produce revolutionary effects, it is critical to evaluate potential risks and problems, such as:

- **Scarring**: Abdominoplasty causes a permanent scar down the lower belly, which can be hidden under clothing but fades over time.
- **Recovery**: Patients may endure swelling, bruising, and discomfort for several weeks after having an abdominoplasty.
- **Potential complications**: Abdominoplasty, like any other surgical surgery, has hazards, including infection.

The Psychological Aspects of Belly Fat

The fight against obstinate belly fat is not only physical; psychological elements that affect our thoughts, feelings, and actions are also intimately linked. Long-term fat loss and lifestyle maintenance depend on an understanding and treatment of these psychological components. We'll look at emotional eating, body image problems, developing a good attitude, goal setting and motivation, and other psychological aspects of belly fat in this chapter.

Affective Eating

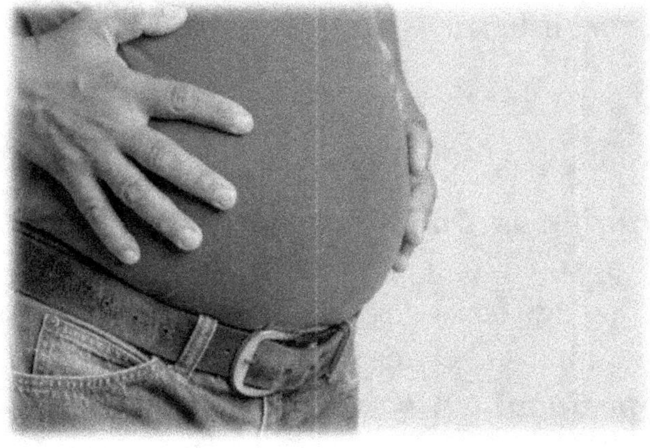

Recognizing Emotional Eating

Emotional eating is the propensity to cope with stress, bad feelings, or other psychological causes by using food. It frequently entails temporarily filling an emotional emptiness or easing emotional pain by eating comfort foods heavy in sugar, fat, and calories.

- ***Stress***: One of the triggers for emotional eating. Emotional eating is a coping mechanism for high levels of stress.
- ***Boredom***: Eating mindlessly to pass the time or divert oneself from unpleasant feelings might result from boredom or emptiness.
- ***Depression or Loneliness***: People who are depressed, lonely, or alone may turn to food for momentary comfort.
- ***Reward or Celebration***: Eating is frequently linked to celebrations or rewards, which encourages overindulgence in reaction to happy feelings or accomplishments.

Tips to Combat Emotional Eating

- ***Mindful Eating***: To improve awareness of physical as opposed to emotional hunger, practice mindful eating by observing hunger signals, enjoying each mouthful, and eating slowly.
- ***Emotional Awareness***: Track patterns and pinpoint underlying emotions by maintaining a food and mood diary to become aware of emotional triggers for eating.

- ***Healthy Coping Mechanisms***: Look into other emotional coping mechanisms include exercise, meditation, journaling, or speaking with a therapist or reliable friend.
- ***Building a Supportive Environment***: Surround yourself with encouraging and accountable others who share your goals.

Body Image Disorders

Behavior Impacted by Body Image

Body image describes how people view, feel, and think about their bodies—including their size, shape, and appearance. Negative attitudes and actions about food, exercise, and self-care that result from poor body image can exacerbate disordered eating patterns and low self-esteem.

Factors Affecting Body Image

- ***Media Influence***: Views of one's own body can be distorted and unhappiness can result from exposure to unrealistic beauty standards in the media, including airbrushed photos and idealized body shapes.
- ***Social Comparison***: Feelings of inadequacy and discontent with one's body can be stoked by comparing oneself to others, in person or on social media.

- ***Past Experiences***: Bad experiences like bullying, criticism, or trauma associated with body image might influence thoughts and feelings about oneself.
- ***Cultural and Societal Norms***: Individual views of body image may be impacted by the differences in cultural standards of beauty and attractiveness between societies and cultures.

Encouraging a Positive Body Image

- ***Self-Compassion***: Emphasize your accomplishments, talents, and attributes that go beyond appearance to cultivate self-compassion and acceptance.
- ***Body Appreciation***: Develop appreciation and thankfulness for the skills, features, and special qualities of your body, whatever its size or shape.
- ***Media Literacy***: Acquire the critical thinking abilities necessary to identify irrational beauty standards presented in the media and question social mores that support body discontent.
- ***Seeking Support***: When things are hard, turn to encourage friends, family, or mental health experts for affirmation, support, and a different viewpoint.

Constructing a Positive Attitude

As attitudes, actions, and results are all influenced by a positive mentality, reaching and maintaining fat loss objectives is impossible without one. Developing a positive attitude is embracing supportive ideas, convictions, and behaviors that encourage and enable people to move forward in the direction of their objectives.

The Advantage of Thinking Optimally
Building a Positive Mindset

- ***Positive Affirmations***: To counter negative thinking, use self-talk or positive affirmations and substitute encouraging and empowering words.
- ***Gratitude Practice***: Make time each day to think back on the things in your life—your body, your health, your relationships, or your accomplishments—for which you are grateful.
- ***Visualization***: See your fat reduction objectives coming to pass by using visualization techniques to see the results you want and the actions required to get there.
- ***Seek Progress, Not Perfection***: Acknowledge a growth mentality by appreciating little accomplishments and growing from disappointments along the road.

Getting Past Self-Limiting Thoughts

Determine which self-limiting ideas—like "I'll never lose weight" or "I'm not capable of change"—may be impeding your ability to reach your fat reduction objectives. Rephrase these convictions as more motivating and doable declarations that encourage self-efficacy and confidence in your capacity for success.

Setting Goals and Motivating Oneself

Building a plan for fat loss achievement requires effective goal setting. Because they are time-bound, relevant, quantifiable, and specified, SMART goals offer a precise structure for establishing goals and monitoring advancement.

A SMART Goal for Fat Loss would be; "*I will lose 1 pound per week by following a balanced diet and exercising for 30 minutes five days a week.*"

Create SMART Goals

- **Measureable**: Using a diary or Smartphone app, "I will track my food intake and exercise activity to monitor progress."
- (Achievable) "I'll start by making little, sustainable changes to my diet and progressively increase the intensity and duration of my workouts."
- **Connected**: "My top goals are to improve my health and lower my risk of chronic diseases, thus losing weight is a reasonable objective."
- **Conservative**: "I will allow for reasonable timeframes and deadlines to reach my target weight of [specific weight] by [specific date]."

Continued Motivation

Sustaining commitment to fat loss goals requires motivation, particularly in trying circumstances or after setbacks. Think on the following approaches to maintain motivation:

- ***Find Your Why***: Whether it's for bettering your health, gaining confidence, or expanding your quality of life, explain why you want to lose stomach fat.
- ***Create Accountability***: Let encouraging friends, family, or a coach hold you accountable and offer encouragement along the road. Share your goals with them.
- ***Applaud Progress***: To keep inspired to keep going, recognize and applaud accomplishments, no matter how little.
- ***Make Any Required Adjustments***: If particular tactics are not working as you had hoped, be adaptable and prepared to change your strategy. Continually be willing to try new things and absorb knowledge from failures.

Summary

In the process of losing weight, psychological elements are quite important since they affect thoughts, feelings, and actions at every stage. Through the treatment of emotional eating habits, development of a healthy body image, development of a resilient mentality, and creation of SMART objectives, people can get beyond psychological obstacles and bring about enduring transformation in their life. Recall that losing weight is about fostering a positive relationship with oneself and accepting the path towards total well-being in addition to physical changes. See case Studies and Success Stories from Real Life in Chapter 8

We explore the specific adventures of people who have effectively overcome obstinate belly fat in this chapter, telling their tales of success, failures, and priceless lessons discovered along the road. These true success stories provide us with understanding of the many routes people have taken to reach their weight loss objectives as well as the recurring themes and tactics that have helped them succeed.

PHASE EIGHT

Belly Fat Loss Personal Journeys

Conquering Emotional Eating

Story of Sarah:

The discovery that Sarah's weight issues were firmly based in emotional eating habits set off her fat loss journey. Sarah used food frequently as a coping technique for stress and anxiety, which resulted in cycles of binge eating and guilt. Resolved to end this harmful cycle, Sarah went to a therapist who assisted her in identifying underlying emotional triggers and creating more constructive coping mechanisms. Sarah discovered how to nourish her body and control her emotions without depending on food by use of mindful eating, self-compassion, and slow lifestyle adjustments. Along with losing extra belly fat, Sarah has now developed a resilience and self-awareness that go well beyond the scale.

Transitioning from a Sedentary to an Active Lifestyle

John's Story

John's path to weight loss started with a health issue that made him rethink his inactive lifestyle. Though John was first unsure of his capacity for change, he resolved to put exercise and healthy living first in his everyday life. John first took baby, doable actions, including going for quick walks and adding more exercise to his daily schedule, and he progressively gained confidence in his capacity to lead an active life. His will to overcome setbacks and remain dedicated to his objectives was fueled by a newfound love of exercise and outdoor pursuits that he eventually discovered. John now not only has a smaller waistline but also feels more alive and empowered since he took charge of his health.

Tips from Prosperous People

The secret is consistency. One recurring theme amongst the many success tales is consistency. Long-term fat reduction success is based on consistency, whether it is in following a nutritious diet, making time for regular exercise, or engaging in mindfulness exercises. Over time, little, durable adjustments done repeatedly produce big benefits and long-lasting habits that promote general well-being.

Attitude Counts

One cannot stress the importance of attitude in reducing body fat. Successful people credit mental and perspective changes as much as physical changes for their accomplishments. People who adopt a positive outlook, reframe failures as chances for personal development, and develop self-compassion can get over challenges and maintain their resilience on the path to weight loss.

The Value of Support Systems

Without the encouragement, accountability, and direction of friends, family, or experts along the way, none of the success stories would have been feasible. Navigating obstacles, maintaining drive, and sharing in successes may all be made much easier with a solid support network.

Accept the Journey

Reaching a particular number on the scale is only one aspect of fat loss; another is accepting the process and the lessons discovered along the way. Every success narrative is evidence of the tenacity, willpower, and development that result from people making the commitment to putting their health and wellbeing first. Through acceptance of the process and celebration of accomplishment, people can bring about significant and long-lasting change in their lives.

Summary

The case studies and actual success stories in this chapter provide anyone starting their own quest to lose obstinate belly fat with inspiration, motivation, and useful information. People can get over challenges, accomplish their weight loss goals, and rewrite their own success stories by adopting consistency, cultivating a positive attitude, and getting help when they need it. Though the path may be difficult at times, the benefits of better health, confidence, and energy make the work well worthwhile.

PHASE NINE

Developing a Personalized Belly Fat Removal Plan

In this chapter, we'll walk you through the steps of developing a personalized belly fat removal plan based on your own needs, preferences, and goals. From assessing your starting point to setting realistic objectives, tracking progress, and making modifications along the way, we'll present practical ideas and resources to assist you in embarking on a successful fat reduction journey.

Understanding your current lifestyle

Begin by evaluating your existing lifestyle, habits, and behaviors about diet, exercise, sleep, stress management, and other things that may contribute to belly fat buildup. Take note of your dietary habits, activity level, sleep quality, stress level, and any pre-existing health conditions or drugs that may have an impact on fat loss.

Body Composition Analysis

Consider conducting a body composition examination to learn about your body fat percentage, muscular mass, and total body composition. This information can help you set more realistic objectives and track your progress than weight or BMI readings alone.

Identifying Areas of Improvement

Determine which aspects of your lifestyle or habits may lead to belly fat buildup, such as excessive calorie consumption, sedentary behavior, poor sleep quality, high stress levels, or unhealthy coping strategies. Understanding these variables will lay the groundwork for designing specific methods to address them.

Setting Realistic Goals

Set SMART (specific, measurable, attainable, relevant, and time-bound) goals for belly fat loss. When defining goals, take into account your present weight, body composition, health status, lifestyle limits, and personal preferences. Aim for slow, sustainable progress rather than quick weight loss, which may be less sustainable in the long run.

Example of SMART goals

- ***Particular***: "I will lose 1 inch from my waist measurement within the next three months."
- ***Measurable***: "I will track my progress by measuring my waist circumference weekly."
- ***Reachable***: "I will aim to create a calorie deficit of 500 calories per day through a combination of diet and exercise."

- ***Significant***: *"Improving my health and reducing my risk of chronic diseases are important priorities for me."*
- ***Time-limited***: *"I will achieve my target waist measurement of [specific measurement] by [specific date]."*

Long-Term and Short-Term Goals

In addition to long-term goals for abdominal fat elimination, break them down into smaller, more manageable milestones or short-term goals. Celebrate each milestone along the road to keep motivated and track your progress properly.

Monitoring food intake

Keep a food diary or use a Smartphone app to monitor your daily food intake, including portion sizes, macronutrient composition, and calorie consumption. Pay attention to your eating habits, causes for overeating, and opportunities to make healthier choices.

Monitoring Physical Activity

Record your workouts, including the type, length, intensity, and frequency. Use a fitness tracker or Smartphone app to track your steps, calories burnt, and progress towards exercise objectives.

Assessing body measurements

Measure your waist circumference, hip circumference, and other pertinent body measurements on a regular basis to monitor changes in belly fat and overall body composition. Take progress images to visually track improvements over time.

Monitoring health markers

Consider measuring additional health indicators such as blood pressure, blood glucose levels, cholesterol levels, and signs of inflammation or metabolic health. Consult a healthcare expert to determine which markers are most relevant to your health goals.

Adjusting Your Plan

Regular Review of Progress

Review your progress on a frequent basis and make adjustments to your plan depending on your body's response and outcomes. Be adaptable and willing to make modifications to your diet, exercise routine, or lifestyle habits if success slows or new challenges emerge.

Seeking Help and Guidance

Don't be afraid to seek help from friends, family members, or health experts who can offer encouragement, accountability, and guidance along the journey. Consider consulting a licensed nutritionist, personal trainer, or health coach to develop a personalized strategy and receive continuous assistance.

Remaining Motivated and Persistent

Maintain your motivation and persistence in the face of adversity or disappointments. Focus on your progress, appreciate your wins, and remember why you started this trip in the first place. Remember that fat loss is a lengthy process that takes patience, persistence, and a dedication to long-term success.

Summary

Creating a personalized belly fat reduction plan is the first step towards attaining your fat loss objectives while also increasing your health and well-being. By assessing your starting place, setting realistic goals, tracking progress, and changing your strategy as needed, you may embark on a successful fat reduction journey personalized to your specific needs and preferences. Remember to remain patient, consistent, and motivated, and don't be afraid to seek help from others when necessary. With focus and determination, you may overcome challenges, break through plateaus, and attain the long-term outcomes you seek.

PHASE TEN

Myths and Misconceptions about Belly Fat

In this chapter, we will debunk popular myths and misconceptions about belly fat, shedding light on inaccurate information, products, and practices that frequently cause confusion and frustration among those looking for fat loss solutions.

Common Myths debunked

Myth 1: **Spot Reduction Is Possible**

One of the most common fallacies regarding belly fat is that you may lose fat in specific parts of the body using exercises or procedures known as spot reduction. However, studies have consistently demonstrated that spot reduction is impossible. While workouts like crunches and leg lifts can strengthen the muscles underlying the fat, they do not burn fat in that specific area. Fat loss happens systemically across the body in response to a calorie shortage, with genetics influencing the order and distribution of fat loss.

Myth 2: **Crash diets cause long-term fat loss**

Crash diets, or severe low-calorie diets, are frequently marketed as quick-fix remedies for rapid fat loss. However, while these diets may produce short-term weight loss, they are neither sustainable nor beneficial for long-term fat loss.

Crash diets can cause muscle loss, nutrient inadequacies, metabolic slowness, and rebound weight gain when normal eating habits are resumed. A healthy, balanced diet, as well as frequent physical activity and lifestyle changes, is required for long-term fat loss.

Myth 3: **Belly Fat Is Just a Cosmetic Concern**

While excess belly fat can certainly have an impact on one's appearance and self-esteem, it's important to understand that belly fat is more than simply a cosmetic issue; it's also a substantial risk factor for a variety of health concerns. Excess visceral fat, in particular, is linked to an increased risk of cardiovascular disease, type 2 diabetes, insulin resistance, metabolic syndrome, and other chronic conditions. Prioritizing fat loss for health reasons, rather than just aesthetics, might provide more motivation and incentive to make long-term lifestyle adjustments.

Myth 4: **Supplements and Waist Trainers are Miracle Solutions**

The weight loss business is inundated with pills, waist trainers, and other goods that promise to reduce belly fat. However, many of these products are not supported by scientific evidence and may possibly be dangerous to health. While certain supplements may have a minor impact on metabolism or hunger, they are not a substitute for a healthy diet and regular exercise. Similarly, waist trainers and corsets can temporarily compress the waistline, but they do not encourage fat loss and may impede breathing and cause discomfort.

Misleading Products and Practices

Avoid goods or programs that make exaggerated or unrealistic claims about belly fat loss, such as "lose 10 pounds in a week" or "melt belly fat without diet or exercise." These claims are frequently misleading and unsupported by scientific evidence. Remember that long-term fat loss involves time, effort, and devotion to healthy lifestyle habits, not quick fixes or magic drugs.

Fad diets and detoxes

Fad diets and detoxes that promise rapid weight loss through extreme restrictions or cleansing regimes may sound enticing, but they are neither sustainable nor effective for long-term fat loss. These diets frequently omit entire food groups, advocate severe calorie restriction, or rely on unproven detoxification procedures that can disrupt metabolism and result in nutrient deficiencies. For long-term outcomes, prioritize balanced nutrition, portion control, and moderation over quick cures.

Too much emphasis on exercise alone

While frequent exercise is an important part of any fat loss program, depending exclusively on exercise without addressing food habits or lifestyle factors may not yield the best outcomes. It is possible to overeat the calorie deficit caused by exercise, particularly if eating habits are not in line with fat loss goals. A comprehensive approach that includes good food, regular physical activity, stress management, and appropriate sleep is essential for attaining and maintaining fat loss.

Pseudoscientific practices

Be aware of pseudoscientific treatments or alternative therapies that promise to reduce belly fat using unconventional methods such as acupuncture, acupressure, sauna suits, or vibrating belts. Some of these activities may provide brief comfort or relaxation, but they are unlikely to result in considerable or long-term fat loss. To achieve the best results, stick to evidence-based solutions supported by scientific research.

Summary

Individuals can make informed decisions and implement evidence-based fat loss tactics by dispelling popular myths and misconceptions regarding belly fat, as well as exposing misleading products and practices. Instead of relying on quick fixes or unreasonable expectations, prioritize good habits, gradual adjustments, and overall health and well-being. Remember that fat loss is a process, not a destination, and success requires persistence, patience, and commitment to long-term lifestyle changes.

Ensuring Long-Term Results

In this chapter, we will look at ways for preserving long-term outcomes after you've met your fat loss goals. From developing sustainable habits to dealing with setbacks and keeping the weight off for good, we'll provide practical information and support to help you successfully navigate the weight maintenance road.

Stay Consistent, Not Perfect

Sustainable Habits

Maintaining long-term success necessitates a shift in thinking from short-term remedies to sustainable habits. Rather than striving for perfection, try for consistency in your daily behaviors about nutrition, exercise, sleep, stress management, and self-care. Accept a balanced approach that allows for flexibility, moderation, and enjoyment in your lifestyle decisions.

Eat a Balanced Diet

Maintain a balanced diet high in whole, nutrient-dense foods such fruits and vegetables, lean meats, whole grains, and healthy fats. Aim to include a diverse range of foods from all dietary groups to guarantee optimal nutritional intake and reduce the risk of nutrient deficits. Maintain a healthy relationship with food by practicing portion management, mindful eating, and paying attention to your body's hunger and fullness cues.

Remain Active and Engaged

Regular physical activity is essential for maintaining weight loss and general health. Find hobbies and workouts that you enjoy and can maintain over time, such as walking, cycling, swimming, yoga, or strength training. Aim for at least 150 minutes of moderate-intensity activity or 75 minutes of vigorous-intensity exercise per week, as well as muscle-strengthening exercises two or more days a week.

Prioritize sleep and stress management

Quality sleep and appropriate stress management are critical for weight management and general health. Aim for 7-9 hours of restful sleep per night, and use relaxation techniques like deep breathing, meditation, yoga, or tai chi to reduce tension and increase relaxation. Prioritize self-care activities that nourish your mind, body, and spirit, such as spending time in nature, interacting with loved ones, or pursuing hobbies and interests.

Dealing with Setbacks

Accept Imperfections

Setbacks and problems are an unavoidable part of the journey, and it is critical to accept imperfections and learn from them without obsessing on them. Instead than seeing setbacks as failures, consider them opportunities for growth, introspection, and course correction. Practice self-compassion and gentleness to yourself, understanding that failures do not determine your worth or growth.

Identifying Triggers and Patterns

When faced with a setback, take the time to discover potential triggers, trends, and underlying causes. Consider your actions, feelings, environment, and external pressures that may have influenced your decisions. Understanding these triggers allows you to build proactive techniques for dealing with them and avoiding future failures.

Focus on Progress, not Perfection

Move your focus from perfection to progress, recognizing tiny successes and gradual improvements along the way. Recognize and acknowledge your efforts, perseverance, and accomplishments, no matter how modest. Celebrate milestones and victories to stay motivated and inspired to keep working towards your long-term objectives.

Keeping the Weight Off

Monitor your progress on a regular basis by keeping track of your weight, body measurements, physical activity, and eating habits. Use this data to keep accountable, spot patterns or areas for improvement, and make changes to your plan as necessary. Regular self-assessment enables you to be proactive and responsive to changes in your body and lifestyle.

Stay connected and accountable

Maintain relationships with helpful friends, family members, and online communities that share your aims and values. Accountability partners can offer encouragement, motivation, and accountability during difficult times, allowing you to stay focused on your long-term goals. Consider joining a support group, doing group exercise classes, or working with a health coach or personal trainer to provide extra accountability and advice.

Celebrate non-scale victories

Shift your emphasis away from the number on the scale and towards non-scale successes and accomplishments related to your overall health and wellness. Celebrate improvements in energy, mood, fitness, strength, mobility, confidence, and overall well-being. Recognize the holistic benefits of your healthy lifestyle practices in addition to weight loss, which will strengthen your dedication to long-term health and vitality.

Summary

To maintain long-term outcomes after attaining your fat loss objectives, you must commit to sustainable behaviors, be resilient in the face of setbacks, and practice constant self-awareness and accountability. By concentrating on consistency, accepting imperfection, and prioritizing holistic well-being, you can successfully traverse the weight management journey and enjoy a lifetime of health, vitality, and happiness. Remember that maintaining long-term outcomes entails more than just arriving at a goal, but also appreciating the journey and lifelong behaviors that promote your health and happiness.

PHASE TWELVE

Resource and Support

In this chapter, we will look at useful tools and sources of assistance to help you on your fat loss journey. These tools, which range from online groups and recommended reading to professional advice from nutritionists and personal trainers, can give you with knowledge, inspiration, and accountability to help you reach your objectives.

Online Communities and Forums

Social Media Platforms

Investigate social media sites such as Facebook, Instagram, Twitter, and YouTube for online communities, groups, and forums focused on weight loss, nutrition, exercise, and wellness. Join organizations or follow accounts related to your goals and values to interact with like-minded people, exchange experiences, ask questions, and find inspiration.

Reddit Subreddits

Reddit has a number of subreddits dedicated to weight reduction, fitness, nutrition, and health, where you can participate in debates, seek advice, and receive support from a wide community of users. Some popular subreddits are r/loseit, r/fitness, r/nutrition, and r/xxfitness (for women).

Fitness Applications and Platforms

Many fitness applications and platforms include community features, challenges, and support networks to connect people who share similar goals. Consider using applications like MyFitnessPal, Fitbit, Strava, or Nike Training Club to track your progress, take part in challenges, and connect with other users for support and accountability.

Suggested Reading and Websites

Books about Fat Loss and Nutrition

Explore a variety of books on fat loss, nutrition, exercise, and healthy living to expand your knowledge and obtain practical insights into attaining your objectives. Some recommended books include "The Obesity Code" by Dr. Jason Fung, "The Complete Guide to Fasting" by Dr. Jason Fung and Jimmy Moore, "Eat to Live" by Dr. Joel Fuhrman, and "The Plant-Based Solution" by Dr. Joel Kahn.

Sites and Blogs

There are numerous websites and blogs dedicated to fat loss, nutrition, exercise, and wellbeing that provide articles, recipes, advice, and tools to help you along your journey. Healthline, Precision Nutrition, the Mayo Clinic, the Harvard Health Blog, and NutritionFacts.org are all trustworthy websites. Explore these websites for evidence-based information and professional advice on a wide range of health issues.

Science Journals and Research

Scientific journals and research articles offer helpful insights and evidence-based advice for anyone interested in learning more about fat loss and nutrition. PubMed, Google Scholar, and Research Gate are examples of websites where you can search for peer-reviewed studies and scholarly papers on your preferred themes.

Professional Support: Dietitians and Personal Trainers

Registered Dietitians and Nutritionists

Consider consulting a qualified dietitian or nutritionist, who may offer personalized nutrition counseling, meal planning, and support based on your specific needs and goals. Dietitians can assist you in developing a healthy eating plan, navigating dietary restrictions or food allergies, and addressing particular issues such as fat loss, metabolism, and overall health.

Certified Personal Trainer

Working with a certified personal trainer can help you gain vital direction, motivation, and accountability on your fitness path. Personal trainers can create personalized training plans, demonstrate proper exercise techniques, and provide support and motivation to help you achieve your fitness objectives safely and effectively. Whether you prefer one-on-one training, small group classes, or online coaching, a personal trainer can give the knowledge and support you require to succeed.

Health Coaches and Wellness Professionals

Health coaches, wellness practitioners, and holistic health specialists provide comprehensive help for achieving general well-being, such as weight loss, stress management, sleep optimization, and lifestyle changes. These specialists take a comprehensive approach to health, addressing the physical, mental, emotional, and spiritual elements of wellness in order to help you attain balance and vitality in all aspects of life.

Summary

By utilizing the resources and support available to you, you may improve your fat reduction journey, learn useful knowledge and insights, and remain motivated and accountable along the way. Whether you're engaging with online groups, researching recommended reading and websites, or seeking professional advice, remember that you're not alone on this path. Accept the help and advice available to you, and continue to invest in your health and well-being to ensure a lifetime of energy and happiness.

Summary

Congratulation for finishing **"Stubborn Belly Fat Remover"**! We have looked at the research, tactics, and useful resources for overcoming obstinate belly fat and reaching your weight loss objectives in this extensive book. From knowing the physiology of belly fat to putting into practice sensible nutrition, exercise, and lifestyle choices, you've learned a great deal that will help you on your path to greater health and vigor.

Remember as you consider the information and techniques in this book that losing weight is about regaining your health, confidence, and general well-being, not just about achieving a number on the scale or fitting into a particular size of clothes. Your body and life can change from the inside out if you give sustainable habits top priority, accept consistency over perfection, and develop a good attitude.

Even although the road to weight loss may be difficult at times, never forget that each step you take forwards you and every barrier you go over is a chance to improve. Despite hardship, be patient, tenacious, and tough, and believe that you can bring about long-lasting change in your life.

Next Actions for You

These are some essential tips to remember as you start your weight loss journey:

- ***Define Realistic Goals***: Define realistic, long-term goals that complement your tastes, values, and way of life. Celebrate every step along the road and keep your attention on progress rather than perfection.
- ***Stay Consistent***: Keep your good habits—diet, exercise, sleep, stress reduction, and self-care—consistent. Over time, little, gradual adjustments done consistently have big benefits.
- ***Get Help***: When you need encouragement, accountability, or direction, don't be afraid to ask friends, family, internet groups, or medical professionals for help.
- ***Continue Learning***: Keep learning about exercise, nutrition, weight loss, and wellbeing. Discover more books, websites, and courses to broaden your knowledge and improve your abilities.

Take Note of Your Body: Attend to the clues, indications, and feedback from your body. Make decisions that feed your body, mind, and spirit; respect your hunger and fullness.

Your Metamorphosis Is Awaiting

Remember that your path to greater health and energy is never-ending when you shut the last chapter of "Stubborn Belly Fat Remover." Accept the difficulties, enjoy the successes, and believe that you can get beyond them and realize your objectives.

One wise decision at a time can change your body and your life. Take advantage of this chance to live your greatest life, release your potential, and give your health first priority.

Ready to advance your fat loss quest, you have to establish your own route going forward. With guts, tenacity, and a firm trust in yourself and welcome it.

Cheers to all of your happiness, health, and prosperity. Best is still to come.

Suggestion

Having given yourself the information, tools, and drive to combat obstinate belly fat, I strongly advise acting right now. Select a strategy or two from each chapter that speak to you and make a commitment to using them regularly. Whether it's changing your diet, getting more exercise, controlling your stress, or consulting a doctor, every constructive action you do advances you towards your objectives.

Recall that losing fat is a marathon, not a sprint. Honor yourself, maintain your attention on your objectives, and have faith in the process. You have all you need for success if you work hard, are persistent, and have this thorough manual at your side.

Never give up, never waver, and let nothing go in the way of your achievement. Start immediately on your path to a happier, healthier, and more self-assured you.

Right now is your moment.

Make it happen.

Synonyms Glossary

Helping you navigate the language used throughout this book and increase your comprehension of the subjects covered, this glossary offers definitions and explanations of important terms and concepts relating to fat loss, nutrition, exercise, and wellbeing.

- ***Measurement of body***: Fat based on height and weight, the Body Mass Index (BMI) is computed by dividing weight in kilograms by height in meter squared. Underweight, normal weight, overweight, and obese are among the categories into which people are divided by BMI.
- ***Calorie Deficit***: The condition where weight loss occurs from calorie expenditure exceeding calorie intake. An often used method for losing weight is to combine diet and exercise to create a calorie deficit.
- ***Macronutrients***: Carbs, proteins and fats are among the nutrients that give energy in the form of calories. Essential to energy generation, metabolism, and general health are these macronutrients.
- ***Metabolism***: The process by which the body uses energy from food to power respiration, circulation, and digestion, among other physiological processes. Age, heredity, physical make-up, and degree of activity can all affect metabolism.

- ***Subcutaneous Fat***: Fat situated under the skin; usually located in the buttocks, hips, and thighs. Insulation and a source of energy, subcutaneous fat is thought to be less dangerous than visceral fat.
- ***Visceral Fat***: Fat kept in the abdominal cavity, around important organs including the pancreas, liver, and intestines. Obesity and type 2 diabetes are among the chronic illnesses linked to excess visceral fat.
- ***Lean Body Mass***: The entire weight of the body—muscle, bones, organs, and fluids—less the fat mass. A vital part of metabolism, strength, and general health is played by lean body mass.
- ***HIIT or high-intensity interval training***: A type of cardiovascular exercise in which intervals of rest or low-intensity exercise alternate with high-intensity exercise. It's well established that HIIT exercises are effective in burning calories, raising cardiovascular fitness, and encouraging fat loss.

Handy Tables and Charts

These tables and charts offer insightful data and visual support for all aspects of your fat reduction journey, from diet and exercise planning to progress monitoring.

- ***The Body Measurement Tracker***: A chart to note measures of important body parts like the circumferences of the thighs, hips, chest, and waist. Monitoring advancement and spotting places for development can be accomplished by keeping an eye on variations in body measurements throughout time.

- ***The Calorie and Macronutrient Calculator:*** A chart or calculator to estimate daily calorie requirements and macronutrient breakdown depending on age, gender, weight, height, degree of exercise, and objectives. You can design a customized diet plan with this tool that is catered to your particular requirements and tastes.
- ***Weekly Meal Planner***: A schedule for breakfast, lunch, supper, and snacks all week long. Making better dietary choices that support your fat loss objectives, saving time and money, and maintaining organization are all made possible by meal planning.
- ***Exercise Log***: A chart or diary used to record workouts together with the kind, length, intensity, and any observations or remarks. Monitoring your development, seeing patterns, and maintaining motivation to maintain your exercise regimen can all be achieved by keeping track of your workouts

Routines for Exercise and Meal Planning

These meal plans and workout schedules provide useful advice and motivation for integrating good eating and exercise into your everyday life, therefore promoting your overall health and fat loss objectives.

- ***Sample Meal Plans***: Weekly or monthly meal plans with wholesome, well-balanced meals and snacks that promote weight loss while supplying vital nutrients and energy. With recipes, serving sizes, and nutritional data, these meal plans could include breakfast, lunch, supper, and snacks.

- **Workout Programs**: Programs are structured workouts suited to various preferences, objectives, and fitness levels. With choices for home or gym-based workouts, these programs may combine strength training, flexibility exercises, aerobic activity, and recovery periods.

- **Progressive Overload**: A strength training tenet that calls for progressively raising the resistance, intensity, or volume of workouts over time to keep the muscles challenged and promote growth and adaptability. Building strength, muscle mass, and endurance as well as preventing fitness plateaus require progressive overload.

- **Rest and Recovery**: The value of rest and recovery—which includes enough sleep, active recuperation, and rest days—in a comprehensive exercise regimen. Body repair and rebuild muscle tissue, restock energy stores, and avoid overtraining and burnout with rest and recovery.

Concluding phase

You may assist your fat reduction journey and reach your goals with the help of the glossary of terms, helpful charts and tables, meal plans, and exercise routines found in this section. Use these resources to more fully grasp important ideas, keep a good record of your development, and put workable success plans into practice.

Recall that long-term success requires consistency, patience, and perseverance; fat loss is a journey rather than a destination. Accept the process, maintain attention on your objectives, and believe that you can bring about long-lasting change in your life and health, vigor and happiness. Let's make every stride towards a happy, healthier you count!

Dear Reader,

Greetings and best wishes as you start your adventure with "Stubborn Belly Fat Remover." I congratulate you for putting your health and well-being first; it takes guts to make the initial move towards good change.

Every word is written with your success in mind, from the most recent scientific data to doable guidance on diet, exercise, and lifestyle modifications.

Beyond the knowledge and tactics, I want you to know that you're not travelling this road by yourself. A community of other readers is walking this road with you, overcoming comparable obstacles and aiming for comparable objectives. We may encourage and support one other along the road, sharing disappointments and enjoying successes.

When you turn the pages of "Stubborn Belly Fat Remover," I want you to read it with an open heart and mind. Knowing that growth chances arise from setbacks and that progress is not always linear, embrace the path with compassion and curiosity.

And I cordially invite you to tell others about your life-changing experience after trial. Someone who might be facing comparable difficulties can find inspiration and drive in your review to make that initial step towards good change.

Your voice counts and others may be motivated to start their own path towards greater health and vigor by your tale. Please think about leaving a review after reading "Stubborn Belly Fat Remover" by *MELISSA J. LEVEY*, so that the world may see your sincere opinion.

With thanks and love, I wish you the very best of luck as you give yourself a trial and you shall be delighted to announce your positive outcome after the trial.

BEST OF LUCK